A CONCISE
MEDICAL DICTIONARY
FOR
HEALTH CARE PRACTITIONERS

About the Author

Dhirendra Verma is a gold meda list from Agra University, from where he received his Master's degree in Science in 1961. He had been a Rockefeller Foundation Research Fellow at the National Institute of Virology in Pune before leaving for Canada in 1963 on a student scholarship to pursue studies at the doctoral level. Subsequently, he was the Head of the Department of Physiology (Faculty of Health Sciences) at the Nova Scotia Institute of Technology in Halifax, Canada.

In 1980, he was invited to Kuwait by its Ministry of Health as a Senior Consultant at the Department of Medical Records and Health Statistics – a position that he held for 22 years, before retiring in 2002. Also, he served the WHO as an individual Consultant contributing extensively to the development, implementation, and training of the ICD (International Classification of Diseases), in the Arabian Gulf Region. For some time he was the Administrative Director of the Al Rashid Hospital – a large private hospital of Kuwait.

Dr. Verma has authored numerous research reports, monographs, and journal articles on relevant contemporary issues in public health.

A CONCISE
MEDICAL DICTIONARY
FOR
HEALTH CARE PRACTITIONERS

DHIRENDRA VERMA, Ph.D.

Former Adviser to the Ministry of Health, Kuwait;
Associate Professor, Deptt. of Health Sciences,
Nova Scotia Institute of Technology, Halifax, Canada;
Rockefeller Foundation Research Fellow,
National Institute of Virology, India;
And
Consultant to WHO & UNESCO

CONCEPT PUBLISHING COMPANY, NEW DELHI-110059

This dictionary is meant to serve as a useful guide to understand health care terms. It should not be relied upon for conclusive medical diagnosis or practice. Neither the publisher nor the author own responsibility for the accuracy of the dictionary for medical diagnosis. All medical matters must be referred to your physician.

ISBN 81-8069-131-4 (H.B.)

First Published 1998

Second Revised Edition 2004

Published and Printed by
Ashok Kumar Mittal
Concept Publishing Company
A/15-16, Commercial Block, Mohan Garden,
NEW DELHI-110059 (India)

Phones : 25351460, 25351794
Fax : 091-11-25357103
E-mail : publishing@conceptpub.com

Dedicated
to
Asha, Sharmila & Mohan,
Resham & Virat

INTRODUCTION

The term “health care” covers an ever-widening range of medical and non-medical work. The members belonging to the health care team come from all walks of life — physicians, dentists, nurses, pharmacists, lab technicians, medical record personnel, epidemilogists, demographers, biostatisticians, community health workers, public health officials, hospital administrators, health care managers, and the like. For effective interaction among these team members it is imperative that they have a thorough understanding of basic terms and concepts so vital to clear communication. Without a common frame of reference we cannot even begin to delineate the problems of health care delivery process, much less carry out a coherent strategy.

One of the greatest barriers to health care workers’ understanding of the current health care scene and its problems and stresses is the language used. Different terms are often applied to the same thing, and many of the terms have multiple meanings. In addition, new terms are appearing daily in health care circles, some with legal and financing developments. Many terms are part of the jargon and slang which are the natural means of communication among insiders. Furthermore, the use of statistical and mathematical techniques so crucial to demographic and epidemiological research as well as to the compilation of routine health statistics, creates a feeling of phobia among those who are not familiar with biostatistical terms, or are not mathematically inclined.

Terminology related confusion prevails among all sectors of health care team *i.e.* physicians, nurses, medical record and laboratory technicians, other paramedical technicians, hospital administrators, and managers of health care systems. Each group suffers in silence while the others use terms that “everybody understands”. In fact, many terms used within one group (physicians or administrators, for example) are not familiar to members of another group and, in the case of new terminology (especially in the area of health care regulation, health care finance, medical statistics and medical jurisprudence), often no one really knows what it means. Recognition of this state of affairs led to the compilation of this dictionary. More specifically, this book endeavours to put in one place definitions that otherwise one would have to look up in several books.

Almost all research studies in health care contain technical terms that non-specialists do not know and, a much greater problem, that they cannot easily look up. What is needed to lower the jargon barrier between readers and research is a handy reference work where students and others can find quick definitions of a wide variety of terms (including various rates and ratios used in vital and health statistics) which are universally applied in health care. I have tried to satisfy this need in this dictionary.

Each definition is intended to present a concept and show how that concept relates to the health care field, and at the same time serve as a quick reference for those already familiar with the concept. The emphasis of the work is on breadth, not depth. In certain instances, however, some depth is necessary to explain the terms ("diagnosis", "foetal death," "prevalence rates," for example); in others, such as the highly technical computations used in biostatistics, no attempt has been made to give detail. Technical terms, such as those from the field of medicine, computers, law and management, are defined simply; they are not intended to be authoritative or to take the place of professional advice.

Many words in the dictionary have more than one meaning. In most cases only the meaning relating to health care is given. For example, "acute" may mean sharp or urgent; the definition given in this work is that relating to disease, meaning one having a sudden onset, sharp rise, and short course. In some instances, a word or phrase has more than one meaning of interest to those in health care. For example "interpolation" has both a statistical and clinical meaning. In these cases, the multiple definitions are listed separately designated as follows :

Interpolation 1. The determination of intermediate values in a series on the basis of observed values.

Interpolation 2. Surgical implementation of tissue.

At the end of the dictionary will be found ten appendices providing internationally accepted ready-reference values for the use of health care practitioners in general and specialized fields. This includes items like medical symbols and formulae used to calculate various morbidity and mortality rates; commonly used medical abbreviations; prefixes and suffixes used in medical terminology; list of essential drugs used throughout the world; trade and generic names of common drugs; common tests and their disease associations; normal range of blood chemistry values; universally accepted immunization schedule for children; and various conversion tables which would be found quite handy by all health care professionals.

The dictionary lays no claim to being complete; new terms appear in the literature almost every day. These will be taken into account in later, updating editions. Both the author and the publisher would be grateful for advice and suggestions.

I should like to thank most sincerely all those people who have so kindly helped me during the compilation of this work, especially Mrs. Susheelamma Varghese for feeding the manuscript into the word-processor and Dr. David Wright, for reading the typescript and for many useful suggestions.

Dhirendra Verma

At the end of the dictionary will be found ten appendices providing internationally accepted ready-reference values for the use of health care practitioners in general and specialized fields. This includes items like medical symbols and formulae used to calculate various morbidity and mortality rates; commonly used medical abbreviations; prefixes and suffixes used in medical terminology; list of essential drugs used throughout the world; trade and generic names of common drugs; common tests and their disease associations; normal range of blood chemistry values; universally accepted immunization schedule for children and various conversion tables which would be found quite handy by all health care professionals.

The dictionary lays no claim to being complete; new terms appear in the literature almost every day. These will be taken into account in later updating editions. Both the author and the publisher would be grateful for advice and suggestions.

I should like to thank most sincerely all those people who have so kindly helped me during the compilation of this work, especially Mrs Susheelamma Varghese for feeding the manuscript into the word-processor and Dr David Wright for reading the typescript and for many useful suggestions.

Dhirendra Verma

CONTENTS

DICTIONARY
OF
HEALTH CARE TERMS

A

Abnormality : 1. The quality or state of being abnormal (deviating from the normal). 2. A malformation.

Abortion : Expulsion from the uterus of the products of conception before the foetus is viable.

Abortion Rate : The estimated annual number of abortions per 1000 women of reproductive age (15-44 years).

Abortion Ratio : The estimated number of abortions per 100 live births in a given year.

Abrasion : A scraped skin surface, such as a skinned elbow which oozes blood.

Abruptio Placentae : Premature breaking off of the placenta, accompanied by haemorrhage, near the end of pregnancy. Causes may be mechanical or toxic.

Abscess : A localized collection of pus in a cavity formed by disintegration of tissues.

Abscissa : The horizontal (X) axis of a graph.

Absolute Alcohol : Ethanol containing not more than 1% by mass of water.

Absolute Values : Numerical values with the signs ignored; thus all absolute values are treated as positive.

Abstinence : Refraining from drug use or from drinking alcoholic beverages whether as a matter of principle or for other reasons.

Abuse (Drug, Alcohol) : A maladaptive pattern of use indicated by continued use despite knowledge of having a persistent or recurrent social, occupational, psychological or physical problem that is caused by the use in situations in which it is physically hazardous.

Acceptance Region : In the theory of hypothesis testing the set of values of the test statistic such that if the test statistic assumes one of these values, the null hypothesis is accepted.

Acceptor : One who adopts a given method of regulating births and/or receives advice through a family planning programme.

Accident : An unpremeditated event resulting in a recognizable injury.

Accomodation : Change in curvature of the lens of the eye to bring objects into sharp focus.

Accountability : Liability to be called to account for action for which one is responsible.

Accreditation : A process of evaluation of the physical, medical, and administrative as well as social and rehabilitative services provided by a health care facility.

Acculturation Difficulty : Slowness or inadequacy in adapting to the demands of a new environment with which the individual could reasonably be expected to cope.

Accuracy : The degree to which variables can be controlled or conform to a standard.

Achievement Test : A psychological test, designed to measure an individual's level of acquired skill or knowledge in a particular field.

Achilles Tendon : The thickest and strongest tendon of the body which binds the muscles of the calf of the leg to the heel bone.

Acholic : Without bile. Clay coloured *acholic stools* indicate some obstructive or other disorders of the liver or bile ducts.

Acidosis : Decreased alkalinity of the blood and other body fluids.

Acne Vulgaris : Common acne. A skin disorder, most conspicuously affecting the face, with pimples and blackheads as the most obvious lesions.

Acromegaly : A disorder of adults due to overproduction of growth hormone by the pituitary glands. The word literally means "giant extremities".

Acrophobia : A morbid fear of heights.

Actinomycosis : An infection or disease caused by fungi which produce unsightly lumpy, pus-draining abscesses, especially common to the face and jaw.

Active Medical Staff : Physicians and dentists who are responsible for the greatest amount of medical practice within the hospital and who perform all significant staff, and administrative functions.

Actuarial Analysis : See *Life Table Analysis.*

Acupuncture : The Chinese practice of piercing specific areas of the body with fine needles for therapeutic purposes.

Acute : Referring to exposure, brief, intense, or short-term. A disease having a sudden onset, sharp rise and short course.

Adaptation : The result of a group of animals or plants being molded by the environmental forces or pressures (climate, altitude, etc.) in a specific region.

Addiction : The state of being surrendered to a habit.

Addition Rule : The probability of obtaining any one of several different outcomes equals the sum of their separate probabilities.

Adhesions : Abnormal sticking together of tissues which should slip or slide freely over each other.

Adipose Tissue : Fatty connective tissue; commonly, the part of the body where fat is stored.

Adjunct Diagnostic Unit : See *Ancillary Unit.*

Adjusted Mean : The mean outcome value that would result if every subject in a group had the same covariate value.

Adjusted Rate : A rate adjusted so that it is independent of the distribution of a possible confounding variable.

Adjustment Disorder : States of subjective distress and emotional disturbance usually interfering with social behaviour and performance, arising in the period of adaptation to a significant life change or a stressful life event.

Adjustment of Rates : A method of correcting for non-comparability with respect to age, race, sex, and so on.

Admission : Formal acceptance, by a health facility, of a patient who is to receive medical or paramedical care while occupying a health facility bed.

Admission Rates : The number of admissions to hospital per unit of population during a specified period of time.

Admitting Officer : Individual responsible for admitting or checking in patients on arrival and discharging or checking out patients as they leave.

Adolescent : The period of years between the beginning of puberty, when the reproductive organs become functionally active, and maturity.

Adrenaline : Proprietary name for *epinephrine,* the hormone produced by the inner portion or medulla of the adrenal gland.

Adult Day Care : Daytime groups or individual service to persons outside their homes by an agency frequently used for the aging or the emotionally disturbed.

Adverse Reaction (Drug) : A toxic physical or psychological reaction to a therapeutic agent (or to a substance of abuse).

Aerobic : Living or functioning in air or free oxygen.

Afterbirth : The placenta and membranes discharged from the uterus a few minutes after the birth of a baby.

Age : Years lived as of last birthday.

Age Adjustment : The application of the age-specific rates in a population of interest to a standardized age distribution in order to eliminate the differences in observed rates that result from age differences in population composition.

Age Specific Fertility Rate : The level of fertility experienced by women of a given age, expressed as a rate.

Age Specific Mortality Rate : The level of mortality experienced by person of a given age, expressed as a rate.

Agencies (Associations, Societies) : Extensions of the individuals who deliver or participate in the delivery of health-care; organized groups.

Agnosia : A loss or impairment of the capacity to recognize objects as a result of perceptual disorder affecting the interpretation of sensory stimuli.

Agonist : A substance that acts at a neuronal receptor to produce effects similar to those of a reference drug.

Agoraphobia : A cluster of phobias embracing fears of leaving home, entering shops, crowds and public places, or travelling alone in trains, buses, or planes.

Agraphia : An ability to express ideas in writing that is unrelated to dysfunction of motor power, speech, or comprehension.

Agreement : Measurement of the extent to which two sets of scores are identical.

AIDS : Acquired immunodeficiency syndrome, an infectious disease caused by a retrovirus, human immunodeficiency virus (HIV).

Albuminuria : Presence in the urine of albumin, a protein like egg white.

Alcoholic : An individual who suffers from alcoholism.

Alcoholism : Chronic continual drinking of alcohol, characterized by impaired control over drinking, frequent episodes of intoxication and preoccupation with alcohol and the use of alcohol despite consequences.

Algol : *ALG*orithmic *O*riented *L*anguage, an international procedure-oriented language.

Algorithm : A finite set of well-defined rules for the solution of a problem in a finite number of steps.

Alkalosis : Increased alkalinity of the blood.

Alkaptonuria : A rare hereditary disorder in which the body is unable to produce enzymes for proper utilization of certain amino acids of protein foods.

Allergen : Any substance capable of producing a state of allergy.

Allergy : The hypersensitive state resulting in an abnormal reaction to a given allergen.

Alopecia : Baldness, loss of head hair.

Alpha Error : See *Type Error*

Alpha Factoring : A method of initial factoring in which the variables included in the analysis are considered samples from a universe of variables.

Alpha Level : The value set by a researcher that specifies the probability of a Type I error (rejecting a true null hypothesis).

Alternative Hypothesis : The opposite of the null hypothesis. Its acceptance means that the results of a study are probably not due to chance.

Alzheimer's Disease : Presenile dementia. A degenerative cerebral disease of unknown aetiology with characteristic neuropathological features, including cortical atrophy.

Amblyopia : Dimness of vision without any organic lesion of the eye.

Ambulance : An automobile that transports the sick or injured—usually at high speed—to a hospital.

Ambulatory : Able to walk; not confined to bed. Patients who make use of outpatient services usually are ambulatory.

Ambulatory Care : All types of health services that are provided on an outpatient basis, in contrast to services provided in the home or to persons who are inpatients.

Ambulatory Surgery : A programme for the performance of elective surgical procedures on patients who are classified as outpatients and typically are released from the surgery centre on the day of surgery.

Amenorrhea : The abnormal absence of menstruation.

Amnesia : Loss or disturbance of memory, attributable to either organic or psychological causes.

Amphetamine : One of a class of sympathomimetic amines with powerful stimulant action on the central nervous system.

Amnion : The innermost of the foetal membranes, forming the "bag of waters" which surrounds and protects the embryo.

Amoebiasis : The state of being infected with amoeba, especially *Entamoeba histolytica*.

Amyotonia : Lack of muscle tone.

Anabolic Steroids : Drugs related to male hormones, sometimes given for anabolic ("upbuilding") action, to stimulate growth, weight gain, strength and appetite.

Anabolism : The "building up" aspects of metabolism, constructive processes of body cells which build complex substances from simpler ones. The opposite of CATABOLISM.

Anaemia : The condition characterized by diminution in the number of circulating red cells and/or their content of haemoglobin.

Anaesthesia : Loss of feeling or sensation.

Anaesthetic : Without feeling. A drug used to induce anaesthesia.

Analeptic : A restorative medicine. A drug that stimulates the central nervous system.

Analgesic : A substance that reduces pain and may or may not have psychoactive properties.

Analog : The representation of numerical quantities by means of physical variables contrasted with digital.

Analysis : A separating or breaking up of any whole into its parts so as to find out their nature, proportion, function, relationship, etc.; a statement of the results of this process.

Analysis of Covariance (ANCOVA) : A statistical procedure designed to control the effects of any variable(s) which is known to be correlated with the dependent variable.

Analysis of Variance (ANOVA) : A statistical test designed to determine if there is a significant difference among several sample means.

Analysis Unit : The unit whose characteristics are tabulated or aggregated to produce statistical results.

Anaphylactic Reaction (or shock) : A severe and sometimes fatal acute allergic reaction in which the outstanding feature is a sudden general circulatory collapse.

Anatomy : The science of the structure or morphology of the body.

Ancillary Unit : An organized unit of a hospital with facilities and personnel to aid physicians in the diagnosis and treatment of patients through the performance of diagnostic or therapeutic procedures.

Ancillary Worker : Health care worker performing in a ancillary unit.

Androgen : A substance that governs the development of the secondary sexual characteristics of the male.

Android : Resembling a man; male-like.

Aneurysm : A blood-filled sac like a thin-walled balloon formed by dilation of artery walls; it is susceptible to rupture and haemorrhage.

Angina Pectoris : Severe substernal pain occurring on exercise and due to coronary artery disease.

Angiography : X-ray of the blood vessels and lymphatic vessels after the injection of a radio-opaque substance.

Angioma : A tumour composed of blood vessels; a class of birthmarks.

Anhidrosis : Abnormal deficiency of sweat production.

Ankylosis : Stiffening or growing together of a joint.

Anomaly : Deviation from normal of an organ or part; abnormality of structure or location.

Anorexia : Loss or absence of appetite. *Anorexia nervosa,* the condition characterized by severe anorexia with loss of weight, usually in young women, and of psychiatric origin.

Anoxia : Oxygen deficiency in organs and tissues and disturbance resulting therefrom.

Antacid : A substance that neutralizes acidity. Usually applied to drugs used to neutralize gastric hyperacidity.

Antagonist : A substance that counteracts the effects of another agent.

Antenatal : Between conception and birth.

Anthrax : A bacterial disease of animals; causative organisms sometimes infect persons who have close contact with raw wool, bristles or hides.

Antibacterial : Destroying or suppressing growth of bacteria.

Antibiotic : A substance produced by micro-organisms which is inimical to other micro-organisms *e.g.* penicillin, streptomycin.

Antibody : A substance produced in the blood and tissues by contact with an antigen, which has the property of destroying the antigen, or the micro-organisms producing the antigen.

Anticoagulants : Drugs which slow up the clotting processes of the blood.

Antidepressant: Psychoactive agents prescribed for the treatment of depressive disorders; also used for certain other conditions such as panic disorder.

Antiemetic : A drug or treatment which stops or prevents nausea or vomiting.

Antigen : A substance that provokes the formation of antibodies.

Antigenic Character : Aspect of chemical arrangement unique to agent and responsible for specificity of immunity resulting from infection.

Antigenicity : Ability to stimulate immune response.

Antihistamines : Therapeutic drugs used in the treatment of allergic disorders and to allay anxiety and induce sleep (because of their sedating effects).

Antinatalist : Policy of government, society, social groups, or religion aimed at slowing population growth.

Antiserum : Serum containing specific antibody.

Antitoxin : A substance which neutralizes a specific bacterial, animal or plant toxin.

Antivenin : An antitoxin to venom, especially snake venom.

Anuria : Total suppression of urine secretion; suggestive of, but not confined to, kidney damage.

Anxiety : The state of being anxious; that is, depressed, worried and apprehensive.

Anxiety State (disorder) : The emotional syndrome, characterized by undue depression, worry and apprehension.

Apex : The summit of a curve.

Aphakia : Absence of the lens of the eye, as after cataract surgery.

Aplastic Anaemia : A grave form of anaemia due to progressive failure of the bone marrow to develop new blood cells.

Apoplexy : A stroke, cerebrovascular accident (CVA); rupture or haemorrhage of vessels into the brain.

Appendectomy : Operation in which the appendix, a small organ in the lower abdomen, is removed.

Appendicitis : Acute inflammation of the appendix.

Applied Research : The application of new knowledge (facts, theories, conclusions) directed towards the accomplishment of a particular requirement.

Arboviruses : A group of viruses transmitted by arthropods (contracted from *ar*thropod-*bo*rn *viruses*).

Area Population : The number of people in a given area (such as nation, province, city, or sample area) in which a specific vital rate applies.

Area Sampling : A method of sampling in which the total area of interest is divided into sub-areas that are then randomly sampled.

Arithmetic Mean : The total of the values of a set of observations divided by the number of observations.

Array : A series of statistical data arranged in a manner to allow for mathematical description or manipulation.

Arrythmia : Any departure from normal rhythm of the heartbeat.

Arteriosclerosis : A thickening or hardening of the walls of arteries leading to a loss of their elasticitiy.

Arthritis (Rheumatoid Arthritis, Osteoarthritis) : Inflammation of joints (involving joint tissues, or bony structures).

Artificial Insemination : Mechanical introduction of semen into the vagina or uterus to induce pregnancy.

Artificial Intelligence : The concept that computers can be programmed to assume some capabilities normally thought to be like human intelligence, such as learning, adaptation, and self-correction.

Asbestosis : Slowly progressing inflammation of the lungs resulting from inhalation of fine asbestos fibres.

Ascariasis : Infestation with species of roundworms which inhabit the large intestine.

Ascites : Painless accumulation of yellowish fluid in the abdominal cavity related to organic disorders.

Asepsis : Absence of infection.

Aspermia : Absence of spermatozoa in seminal fluid.

Asphyxia : The condition characterized by lack of oxygen, and excess of carbon dioxide, in the tissues, and usually due to interference with respiration.

Aspiration : Removal of fluids or gases from a body cavity by suction.

Assay : Determination of the amount of a particular constituent of a mixture, or of the potency of a drug.

Assessment : An objective determination of the degree to which test results satisfy specified test objectives.

Associate Medical Staff : Physicians or dentists who are new to the staff and are being considered for advancement to the medical staff.

Association : Relationship between variables.

Assumption : A fact or relationship thought to be true but not proven or verified.

Asthma : A respiratory disorder marked by recurrent attacks of paroxysmal dyspnoea, with wheezing due to spasmodic contraction of the bronchi.

Astigmatism : Distortion of vision resulting from imperfect curvature of cornea or lens of the eye.

Asymptotic : When a line on a graph continually approaches but never reaches the X axis.

Ataxia : Loss of muscle coordination; groups of muscles cannot be brought into concerted action.

Atelectasis : A retracted or collapsed state of the lung which leaves all or part of the organ airless.

Atherosclerosis : Degeneration of blood vessels caused by a deposit of fatty materials along the lining of the wall of a blood vessel.

Atresia : Closure or failure of development of a normal opening or channel in the body.

Atrophy : Washing away or shrinking in size of a previously normal organ, tissue or part.

Attack Rate : Number of persons attacked with a specific disease per 100 or 1000 at risk, *i.e.*, in the population groups specified.

Attributes : Characteristics that can be expressed in qualitative classifications.

Audiologist : A person skilled in audiology (the science of hearing), including the rehabilitation of those whose impaired hearing cannot be improved by medical or surgical means.

Audiometer : An electrical instrument used in measuring acuity of hearing for sounds of different frequencies.

Audit : An examination or review that establishes the extent to which a condition, process, or performance conforms to predetermined standards or criteria.

Autism : The condition of being dominated by subjective, self-centered trends of thoughts or behaviour which are not subject to correction by external information.

Autoclave : An automatically controlled apparatus for sterilization by means of steam.

Autocorrelation : The internal correlation between members of a time series separated by a constant interval of time.

Auto-immune Disease : Disease caused by immunologic response to a host's own tissue antigen.

Autoimmunity : The process whereby an individual develops or acquires antibodies to his own tissues.

Autolysis : Self-digestion of tissues in the body by enzymes produced by the cells of the tissue concerned.

Automation : The investigation, design, development, and application of 'methods' of rendering processes automatic, self-moving, or self-controlling.

Autopsy : Post-mortem examination (examination of a body after death); necropsy.

Autoregression : A regression structure in which lagged response values assume the role of the independent variables.

Auxillary Unit : See *Ancillary Unit.*

Auxiliary Worker : See *Ancillary Worker.*

Average : A measure of central tendency or central location of data.

Average Annual Rate of Change : Geometric rate of per cent change which assures that a variable increases or decreases at the same rate during each year between the two time periods.

Average Bed-Duration : The total length of bed duration (in days) for patients who have been discharged within a given period, divided by the number of discharges in the period.

Average Cost : The cost per unit of output (total cost divided by total number of units of outputs). Also known as *unit cost.*

Average Daily Census : Average number of inpatients present each day for a given period of time.

Average Length of Stay (ALOS) : The average length of hospitalization of inpatients discharged during the period under consideration.

Aversion Therapy : A treatment that suppresses undesirable behaviour by associating a painful or unpleasant experience with the behaviour.

Avulsion : The forcible tearing away of a part.

Axilla : The armpit.

Axon : A single long fine fibre which conducts impulses away from the body of a nerve cell.

Azoospermia : Absence of sperm in the semen.

B

Babinski Sign : Upward movement of the big toe and downward movement of other toes when the sole of the foot is stroked; an indication of nervous system disorder.

Backward Induction : The method used in solving a decision problem under uncertainty by means of a decision tree diagram.

Bacteremia : The presence of living bacteria in circulating blood.

Bacteria : Tiny, colourless, single-celled organisms of the vegetable kingdom.

Bactericidal : Causing the death of bacteria.

Bacteriostatic : Inhibiting growth or multiplication of bacteria; an agent that so acts.

Bagassosis : Chronic inflammation of the lungs caused by inhalation of bagasse, the material left from crushed sugar cane after its juices have been extracted.

Bar Chart (or Bar Graph) : The depiction of relationships among elements. The rectangle is the essential representation of the area of the bar.

Barbiturates : Derivatives of barbituric acid, used as hypnotics.

Barium Meal : A suspension of insoluble barium sulphate in water, swallowed in preparation for a "G.I. series".

Basal Metabolic Rate (B.M.R.) : The speed at which a body at rest uses oxygen to consume the calories in food.

Basic Health Services : A network of institutions run by the government as part of the country's administrative system that provides certain indispensable medical care and preventive services to individuals.

Basic Research : Efforts directed towards the increase of knowledge to science, the primary aim of the investigator being a fuller knowledge, or understanding of the subject under study.

Bayes' Rule/Bayes' Theorem : A formula used to calculate conditional probability of one event from the conditional probability of the other event.

Bayesian Statistics : An area that deals primarily with topics such as Bayesian decision theory, Bayesian estimation, and Bayesian regression analysis.

B.C.G. : *B*acillus of *C*almette and *G*uerin; a vaccine which gives immunity to tuberculosis for a variable time.

B.E.A.M. : Abbreviated form of *b*rain *e*lectrical *a*ctivity *m*apping. Computer-enhanced analysis and display of electro-encephalographic and evoked response studies.

Bed *:* One bed in a 24-hour section for treatment of a patient within a health care facility.

Bed Count (Bed Capacity, Bed Complement) : The number of available facility inpatient/resident beds, both occupied and vacant, on any given day.

Bed Count Day : A unit of measure denoting the presence of one inpatient/resident bed (either occupied or vacant) set up and staffed for use in one 24-hour period.

Bed Count Days (Total) : The sum of inpatient/resident bed count days for each of the days in the period under consideration.

Bed Day : 24 hours in which a 24-hour patient has received treatment.

Bed Duration : Number of bed days for a 24-hour patient, the date of admission, but not the date of discharge is included; at least 24 hours.

Bed Occupancy Ratio (B.O.R.) : The proportion of beds occupied, defined as the ratio of service days to bed count days in the period under consideration (synonymous terms: per cent occupancy, occupancy per cent, occupancy ratio).

Bedpan : A shallow vessel used for defecation or urination by patients confined to bed.

Bedsore : An area of inflamed or ulcerated skin, overlying bony prominences in patients confined to bed for long periods.

Bed Turnover Interval : The average time a bed remains empty between patients : calculated by dividing the total of vacant bed days during a year by the number of patients leaving hospital (by discharge, transfer or death) during that year.

Bed Turnover Rate (or Throughput) : The numbers of times a bed, on the average, changes occupants during a given period of time : calculated by dividing the number of separations (transfers, discharges, deaths) by the mean number of available beds.

Bed Utilization Statistics : Statistics dealing with resource utilization measures in a hospital such as A.L.O.S. (Average Length of Stay). B.O.R. (Bed Occupancy Ratio), T.O.R. (Turnover Rate) and T.O.I. (Turnover Interval).

Behaviour Disorders : Disorders of abnormal behaviour and emotions which are less severe than psychoses but more resistant to treatment than transient situational disturbances.

Behaviour Therapy : Treatment of psychological disturbance through an approach directed at unlearning faculty or limiting behaviour or response, *e.g.* phobias.

Behavioural Sciences : The study of human development, values, experiences, activities, interpersonal relationships, such as psychology, psychiatry, sociology, political science, and ethology.

Beliefs : Ideas and concepts moulded by education, religion and parental influence which play a major role in opinion and behaviour.

Bell-shaped Distribution : A term used to describe the shape of the normal (gaussian) distribution.

Bell's Palsy : Paralysis of the facial nerve, usually temporary.

Benefit/Cost Ratio : The ratio of net present value of measurable benefits to costs: used to determine the economic feasibility or success of a programme.

Benefit/Risk Ratio : The ratio of benefit to risk in the use of a drug; a means of expressing a judgement concerning the role of the drug based on efficacy and safety data.

Benign : Mild, usually the word means that a tumour is not cancerous.

Benzodiazepines : The generic name for a group of compounds (Valium, Librium, Serax, Ativan, Mogadon, etc.) used for the symptomatic relief of anxiety and insomnia.

Bereavement : Feeling of deprivation, desolation and grief at the loss of a loved one.

Beriberi : A deficiency disease, chiefly the result of a deciciency of thiamine (Vitamin B_1) in the diet.

Bernoulli Process : A random process that yields an either/or outcome on each trial with known probability of occurrence, and results from statistically independent trials.

Bestiality : Sexual relations between a human being and an animal.

Beta Level, Beta Error : The probability of committing a Type II error.

Between-Group Variance : In analysis of variance, differences among the means of the various groups.

Bias : The occurrence of some influence in a study that tends to give an advantage or disadvantage to one or more sub-groups in the study.

Biased Sample : A non-randomly selected sample such that all possible samples from a population do *not* have an equal chance of being selected.

Bile : A brownish-yellow fluid secreted by liver and stored in the gallbladder.

Bilirubin : The principal pigment of bile; a reddish substance derived from the breakdown of haemoglobin.

Bimodal Distribution : A distribution that has two pronounced peaks when graphed as a frequency polygon.

Binomial Measurement : A measurement in which the individual is placed in one of two mutually exclusive categories (*e.g.* heads or tails, male or female).

Bioassay : The quantitative evaluation of the potency of a substance by assessing its effects on tissues, cells, live experimental animals, or humans.

Bioavailability : The rate and extent of absorption of a drug from a dosage form as determined by its concentration/time curve in the systemic circulation or by its excretion in urine.

Biofeedback : The use of instrumentation to increase subjective awareness of bodily functions (muscle tension, blood pressure, heart rate, temperature, etc.) in order to treat anxiety, migraine, hypertension, headaches, etc.

Biological Clock : Physiological mechanism that controls periodic changes or rhythms in various physical and behavioural functions. *e.g.* body temperature or blood pressure.

Biological Rythms : Cyclical variations in physiologic and biochemical function, level of activity and emotional state.

Biometry : The application of statistical methods to the study of numerical data based on biological observations and phenomena.

Biopsy: The examination of living tissue removed from the body for diagnostic purposes.

Biostatistics : Application of statistics to biological (including medical) problems.

Bipolar Disorder : A mood disorder in which there are episodes of both mania and depression, and in which the patient's mood and activity levels are significantly disturbed (formerly called manic-depressive psychosis).

Birth Certificate : Official, legal document recording details of a live birth, usually comprising name, date, place, identity of parents, and birth weight.

Birth Cohort : A birth cohort consists of all persons born within a given period of time, such as a year.

Birth Order : Rank of each live child a woman has born.

Birth Rate : The number of live births in a geographical area during a time period divided by the estimated population of the area — usually expressed per 1000 persons per year.

Birth Weight : The first weight of the foetus or newborn obtained after birth.

Low Birth Weight : Less than 2500 g

Very Low Birth Weight : Less than 1500 g

Extremely Low Birth Weight : Less than 1000 g.

Bisexual : Equally attracted to the two sexes : hermaphrodite.

Bit : Acronym for *b*inary dig*it* : Either of the digits 0 and 1 when it is used as a signal in computing.

Bivariate Distribution : A joint distribution of two variables, wherein scores on one variable are normally distributed for each score value of the other.

Bivariate Regression : A statistical method for obtaining a straight line that describes the relationship between two variables.

Blackout : Temporary loss of consciousness.

Blepharitis : Inflammation of the eyelids, usually associated with bacterial infection or allergy.

Blind Spot : A small spot on the retina, where the optic nerve enters, which is insensitive to light.

Blind Study : An experimental study in which subjects do not know the treatment they are receiving; investigators may also be blind to the treatment subjects are receiving.

Blood Alcohol Level (B.A.L.) : The concentration of alcohol (ethanol) present in blood—usually expressed as mass per unit volume.

Blood Bank : Storage place for bottled (or plastic-bagged) human blood to be used in transfusions.

Blood Count : The number of red or white blood cells in a cubic millimetre of blood.

Blood Donor : One who gives blood for therapeutic purposes.

Blood Group : One of the genetically determined series (A, B, AB, O) into which the blood is divided and which is of great importance in blood transfusion and medico-legal jurisprudence.

Blood Transfusion : Injection of properly cross-matched human blood into a patient.

Body Image : One's sense of self and one's body as presented to others.

Bonding : Development of an attachment between persons in a relationship whose identities are significantly affected by their mutual interactions.

Boolean Algebra : A process of reasoning, or a didactic system of theorems using a symbolic logic, and dealing with classes, proportions, or on-off circuit elements.

Booster Shot : Injection of a vaccine or immunizing agent given some time after an original vaccination, to enhance its effectiveness.

Botulism : A fatal form of food poisoning induced by contamination of food by *Clostridium botulinum.*

Box-and-Whisker Plot (or Box Plot) : A pictorial description of the median, first and third quartiles, and lowest and highest scores of one or more groups.

Bracketing : The operation of combining categories or ranges of values so as to produce a small number of categories. Sometimes referred to as "collapsing or grouping".

Bradycardia : Abnormal slowness of the heartbeat, with a pulse rate of less than 60 per minute.

Braille : The system of printing by means of raised points to enable the blind to read by touch.

Brain Imaging : Any technique that permits the in vivo visualization of the central nervous system (*e.g.* CT, MRI, PET, RCBF, BEAM).

Brain Washing : Techniques including indoctrination, repeated suggestions and mental exhaustion to produce deliberate transformation of attitudes or personality in pursuance of some political or other non-therapeutic aim.

Breech Delivery : Presentation of an infant's buttocks instead of the head at the outlet of the birthcanal.

Bronchitis : Inflammation of the linings of lung's bronchial tubes.

Brucellosis : An infectious disease transmitted from goats, sheep or cows to man, by contact with cattle or consumption of raw milk products.

Bruxism : Grinding of the teeth, occurs unconsciously while awaken or during stage 2 sleep. May be secondary to anxiety, tension, or dental problems.

Bubonic Plague : Plague marked by swelling of the lymph nodes (buboes) : spread by infected rats and other rodents.

Budget Surplus : Central government current and capital revenue and official grants received, less expenditure and net government lending.

Buggery : Usually refers to anal intercourse, either hetero- or homosexual, but in law refers to both sodomy and bestiality (sexual contact with an animal).

Bulimia Nervosa : Repeated bouts of overeating and an increasing preoccupation with the control of body weight, leading to a pattern of overeating followed by vomiting or use of purgatives.

Bunion : Enlargement and thickening of the big joint of the big toe, bending the big toe towards the little toe.

Burn-out : A state of physical or emotional exhaustion in response to the stress of unrelenting performance demands stemming from the individual's occupation.

Bursa, Bursitis : A sac between opposite surfaces that slide past each other, the inflammation of which is called *bursitis.*

Bus : A common pathway shared by signals from several components of the computer.

Byte : A group of adjacent bits commonly 4, 6, or 8, operating as a unit for storage and manipulation of data in a computer.

C

Cachexia : Profound weakness, emaciation, general ill health, resulting from serious disease such as cancer.

Caesarean Section : Delivery of a child by surgical opening of the uterus.

Caesarean Section Rate : The total number of caesarean sections performed in a period divided by the total number of deliveries in the period including caesarean section, multiplied by 100.

Calcification : The process of depositing of lime salts in the tissues.

Calculus : A stone found mainly in ducts or hollow organs, such as the gallbladder, bile duct, bladder and ureter.

Callisthenics : Gymnastics aimed at producing beauty and grace of movement.

Callus : A patch of hard, thickened skin, usually on hands or feet; a protective reaction to pressure or friction.

Cancer : A term used rather loosely, usually as an alternative to carcinoma, but it is also used to denote any malignant new growth.

Cannabis : A generic term used to denote the several psychoactive preparations of the marijuana (*hemp*) plant, *Cannabis sativa.* They include marijuana leaves (*bhang*), flowering shoot (*ganja*), and resinous matter collected from the plant (*charas*). *Hashish* is a powdered and sifted form of charas.

Cannula : A hollow tube for insertion into a body passage or cavity.

Capital Expenditure : Expenditure on land, buildings, and initial equipment and supplies to establish or extend health facilities such as health centres, laboratories and hospitals.

Carbuncle : An acute circumscribed inflammation of the skin and subcutaneous tissues, usually due to *Staphylococcus aureus.*

Carcinogen : A cancer-producing agent or factor.

Carcinogenesis : The production of carcinoma in the living tissues.

Carcinoma : A malignant tumour of epithelial cells which spreads locally and metastasizes in a completely uncontrolled manner.

Cardiology : Medical specialty focusing on heart problems. A physician who practices this specialty is a cardiologist.

Cardiovascular : Pertaining to the heart and blood vessels.

Care : Management of, responsibility for, or attention to the safety and well-being of another or other persons.

Care Unit : An organizational entity of a health care facility. Facilities are organized both physically and functionally into units to provide care.

Caries : A process of gradual decay of bone and teeth.

Carminative : A drug that facilitates eructation (belching).

Carriers (Chronic) : Healthy persons harbouring and excreting an infectious agent (for a long period or indefinitely).

Carryover Effect : A confounded effect that results when a new treatment is given while the effects of previous treatments are still present.

Case : Another name for patient. Each patient is considered a medical case to be diagnosed and treated.

Case-Control Study : An hypothesis-testing in which data are collected from (1) patients with the disease being explored, and (2) an appropriate sample of control subjects (who may be matched for sex, age, and other attributes).

Case-Fatality Rate : The number of patients dying from a specific condition, divided by the number developing the condition—usually expressed per 1000 affected persons.

Case Mix : A means of classifying hospital patients to provide a common basis for comparing cost effectiveness and quality of care across hospitals.

Case Mix Index (CMI) : A single number which compares the overall complexity of the hospital's medicare patients to the complexity of the average for all hospitals in the U.S.

Castration : Removal of the testicles or ovaries,

Cataract : Partial or complete opacity in the lens of the eye.

Catchment Area : Region, which may be well- or ill-defined, from which the clients of a particular health facility are drawn.

Cathartic : Having a purgative or purifying action. A purgative.

Catheter : A tube for passage through the urethra or other canals for purposes of drainage or withdrawing fluids.

Cause-Specific Mortality-Rate : The number of deaths from a specific cause divided by the estimated mid-year population at risk — expressed per 1000 persons per year.

Cautery : Application of heat or a chemical to destroy tissue.

CCU : Initials for *C*oronary *C*are *U*nit or *C*ardiac *C*are *U*nit, a hospital unit for constant monitoring and care of heart patients.

Celiac Disease : A hereditary disorder in which the small intestine is unable to aborb fat from foods.

Cell : In two-way ANOVA, any combination of levels for two factors. **Cell mean :** The mean of all the observations in a cell. **Cell size :** The number of observations in a cell. **Cell S.D. :** The standard deviations of all the observations in a cell. In biology, a very small unit of protoplasm, usually with a nucleus, cytoplasm, and a cell wall.

Cellulitis : Inflammation in cellular tissue, especially subcutaneous tissue.

Censored Observation : An observation whose value is unknown, generally because the subject has not been in the study long enough for the outcome of interest, such as death, to occur.

Census : 1. The number of inpatients present in a health care facility at any one time. 2. An official, usually periodic, count of population and recording of economic status, age, sex, etc.

Centerline : The line midway between the control limits on a control chart. It is the grand average of all the sample statistics plotted on the control chart.

Central Limit Theorem : The mathematical theorem that states that the sampling distribution of means approaches a normal curve as the sample size increases.

Central Processing Unit (CPU) : A unit of a computer that includes circuits controlling the interpretation and execution of instructions.

Central Tendency : A statistic that indicates where in the distribution scores tend to bunch. The mean, median, and mode are common measures of central tendency.

Cerebral Palsy : A group of chronic non-progressive disorders of the brain present from birth or acquired during the developmental period and characterized by bilateral disturbances of motility.

Cerebrovascular Accident (CVA) : A sudden disturbance of cerebral function attributable to vascular disease, principally thrombosis, haemorrhage, or embolism.

Cerumen : Ear wax. The secretion of the ceruminous glands of the external auditory meatus.

Cervical : Pertaining to the neck or the cervix of an organ.

Chadwick's Sign : A blue discolouration around the entrance to the vagina and on the neck of the uterus; an early indication of pregnancy.

Chance Agreement : A measure of the proportion of times two or more raters would agree in their measurement or assessment of a phenomenon.

Chancre : The primary lesion of syphilis; a hard sore or ulcer at the site where syphilis germs gained entrance to the body.

Chart : Folder on each patient where the doctor and the nurse record all forms of treatment, all measurements of vital signs, and so on.

Check Digit : A single digit, derived from a multi-digit number such as a case identification number, that is used as a screening test for transcription errors.

Chemoprophylaxis : Use of a chemical, including antibiotics, to prevent the development of an infection or the progression of an infection to active manifest disease.

Chemotherapy : Use of a chemical to cure a clinically recognizable disease or to limit its further progress.

Child Abuse : Maltreatment of a child, whether by neglect or by intentional exploitation or injuring.

Child Death Rate : The number of deaths of children aged 1-4 years in a given year per 1000 children in this age-group.

Chip : A small computer device containing memory space and machine software.

Chi-Square Distribution : A theoretical sampling distribution of chi-square values. The shape of the chi-square distribution changes as a function of the degrees of freedom.

Chi-Square Statistic : A measure of the level of significance between a set of *observed* and *expected* values.

Chi-Square Test : A statistical method used to test whether the classification of data can be ascribed to chance or to some underlying law.

Cholecystectomy : Operation for removal of the gallbladder.

Cholecystitis : Inflammation of the gallbladder.

Cholelithiasis : The presence of gallstones in the common bile duct.

Cholera : A serious acute intestinal disease, characterized by the sudden onset of severe diarrhoea, and due to *Vibrio cholerae.*

Cholesterol : A steroid alcohol, normally present in the blood to the extent of 150 to 250 mg per 100 ml which is essential for the many body processes.

Chromosome : One of the rod-shaped bodies in the nucleus of a cell that carry the genes or factors of inheritance.

Chronic : 1. Referring to a health-related state, being of long duration. 2. Referring to exposure, prolonged or long-term, often with specific reference to low intensity.

Civil Registration : The traditional method of registration of births and deaths, providing both legal documentation of each vital event and statistical records for the compilation of vital statistics.

Circumcision : Removal of the prepuce in the male, or the labia minora in the female.

Cirrhosis (Liver) : Disease associated with a great increase of fibrous tissue throughout the liver (usually following acute destruction of liver cells).

Class : One of the intervals into which the entire range of the variable has been divided.

Class Frequency : The number of observations in each class.

Class Interval : The difference between two consecutive lower class limits in a frequency distribution.

Class Limits : The true values at the beginning and end of each class.

Class Marks : The variable values that demarcate each class.

Class, Social : A method of socially stratifying populations, *e.g.* according to education, income, or occupation.

Classical Statistics : An area that deals primarily with topics such as statistical inference and regression analysis.

Classification of Diseases : Arrangement of diseases into groups having common characteristics; useful in the presentation of morbidity and mortality data for comparative purposes.

Claudication : Lameness, limping. Intermittent claudication may be a symptom of obliterative arterial disease.

Claustrophobia : Abnormal fear of enclosed spaces.

Cleft Lip, - Palate : Congenital malformation of structures of the lip, palate, or both, which fail to fuse properly during foetal development.

Clinic Outpatient : An outpatient who is admitted to a clinical service of the clinic or hospital for diagnosis or treatment on an ambulatory basis.

Clinical Service : A unit of medical staff responsibility (*i.e.* Cardiology), a unit of inpatient beds (*i.e.* general medical), or even a group of discharged patients with related diseases or treatments (*i.e.* orthopaedic surgery).

Clinical Syndrome : Combination of symptoms and physical signs which accompany disease.

Clinical Trial : A study that evaluates the effectiveness of one or more interventions in human subjects by comparing the intervention group(s) with a suitable control group.

Clone : The asexual progeny of a single cell.

Closed Birth Interval : Interval between two successive births.

Clot : A semi-solid mass of coagulated blood, lymph, or other body fluid.

Clubfoot : A foot twisted out of shape so that the sole does not rest flat on the floor when standing.

Cluster Sampling : A sampling scheme in which each unit selected is a group of persons (all persons in a city block, a family, etc.) rather than an individual.

Coastal Cities : Coastal area is defined as a zone no more than 60 kilometers inland.

Cobol : *C*ommon *B*usiness *O*riented *L*anguage. A business data processing language.

Coccus : A sphere-shaped bacterium.

Cochlea : A small, snail-shell like structure of the inner ear, lined with fine hair and nerve endings which are the essential organs of hearing.

Codes : Symbolic abbreviations that allow information to be categorized into succinct forms for ease of storage and use.

Coding : A numerical assignment that provides an organized approach to data retrieval.

Coefficient of Determination : A squared correlation coefficient which indicates the amount of variation of Y scores accounted for by the variation of X scores. An estimate of common or shared variance.

Coefficient of Variation (CV) : The standard deviation divided by the arithmetic mean (generally multiplied by 100); used to obtain a measure of relative variation.

Cohort : Group of people (usually 100,000) born at the same time interval, such as a year.

Cohort Study : Investigation of a group of individuals, who share some common characteristic, and follow-up of those individuals over a period of time.

Colic : Pertaining to the colon. Spasmodic griping pain in the abdomen.

Colitis : Inflammation of the colon.

Colostomy : The surgical creation of an artificial anus in the colon.

Colostrum : The first milk from the mother's breasts after the birth of her baby.

Colpectomy : Surgical removal of the vagina.

Column Per cent : In a cross-tabulation, the result of dividing a cell frequency by the number of cases in the column.

Coma : A state of profound unconsciousness, from which the patient cannot be aroused.

Combat Fatigue : A state of emotional and physical exhaustion precipitated by the experience of combat.

Commercial Energy : Commercial forms of primary energy — petroleum products, natural gas, solid fuels, and primary electricity —all converted into oil equivalents.

Commodities : In a family planning programme, contraceptive materials, such as pills, IUDs, condoms, used in the programme.

Common Factor : Unmeasured (or hypothetical) underlying variable which is the source of variation in at least two observed variables under consideration.

Common (or shared) Variance : See *Coefficient of Determination.*

Communality : The variance of an observed variable accounted for by the common factors.

Communicable Disease : An illness due to an infectious agent which arises through transmission of that agent from an infected person or animal to a susceptible host, through an intermediate host or vector.

Communicable Period : The time during which an infectious agent may be transferred from an infected person to another person.

Communicability (Period of) : Time during which a patient with an infectious disease is a potential source of infection for other persons.

Community : A group of individuals organized into a unit, or manifesting some unifying trait or common interest. The locality or catchment area population for which a service is provided.

Community Health Worker : Trained health workers who live within the community and work with the health and development workers as a team.

Community Hospital : The most common type of hospital, offering general, short-term care to acutely or severely ill patients.

Commuter : In migration studies, a person who journeys regularly between work and home (not a migrant).

Comorbidity : A pre-existing condition that will, because of its presence with a specific principal diagnosis, cause an increase in the patient's length of stay by at least one day in 75% of the cases.

Compatibility : The ability to transfer computer programmes and computer readable data from one hardware system to another without losses, changes, or extra programming.

Compliance (drug) : Faithful adherence by the patient to the prescriber's instructions.

Complication : A condition that arises during the hospital stay that prolongs the patient's length of stay by at least one day in 75% of the cases.

Component : Any of the simple or compound parts of some complex thing or concept.

Compound Fracture : One in which the broken bone breaks through the skin or into an open wound.

Comprehensive Health System : A system that includes *all* the elements required to meet *all* the health needs of the population.

Compulsory Education : The existence of laws that stipulate that children, unless exempted, must attend a certain number of grades, between designated ages.

Computer : A data processor that can perform substantial computation without intervention by a human operator during a run.

Computer Package : A set of statistical computer programmes for analyzing data (*e.g.* SPSS).

Computer Programme : A set of instructions stored in the computer which directs it to perform a specific process.

Concept : A complex of ideas so united as to portray a large general idea.

Conception : 1. The act of becoming pregnant. 2. The act of forming ideas.

Concordance : In harmony; or agreement.

Concurrent : Occurring at the present time. A study of currently occurring conditions is a concurrent study.

Concussion : Violent jarring, shocking, shaking or the resulting condition.

Condition : A health condition is a departure from a state of physical or mental well-being.

Conditional Distribution : In regression, the spread of Y scores for a given X score.

Conditional Probability : The probability that A will occur given that B has occurred.

Condom : A sheath worn over the penis during coitus to prevent conception.

Confidence Interval/Confidence Limits : A range of values within which a researcher can state with a certain degree of confidence (often with 95% confidence) that the true but unknown population value will fall.

Confidentiality : Status accorded to data or information which is sensitive and must be protected against improper use and disseminated only to individuals authorized to have it.

Configuration : The particular choice of hardware and its connections making up a computer system.

Conformance : Meeting standards; state of having met standards.

Confounding : A situation in which there is more than one possible explanation for a particular study outcome.

Confounding Variable : An uncontrolled variable that systematically co-varies with the independent variable.

Confusion : A state of impaired consciousness associated with acute or chronic cerebral organic disease.

Congenital Malformation : Defect occurring during embryonal or foetal development.

Conjunctivitis : Inflammation of the conjunctiva (the transparent membrane lining the eye and eyelids).

Consanguinity : Blood relationship.

Consent : Concurrence of wills; voluntary yielding of one's will to the proposition of another.

Consistency : Repeated similar behaviour of data.

Constant : A numerical value that is exactly the same for all cases or subjects; the converse of *variable.*

Consultation : The response by one health care professional to the request by another health care professional to provide recommendations and/or opinions regarding the care of a particular patient.

Consultation Ratio : The number of general practitioner consultations for a condition in relation to the size of the practice list and a specified period of time.

Consumer : Recipient of product or service. In health care, thought to have fewer connotations of subservience than the analogous terms *patient* and *client.*

Consumer Price Index (CPI) : A monthly measure of the average change in the prices paid by urban consumers for a fixed market basket of goods and services. The medical care component of CPI shows trends in medical care prices based on specific indicators of hospital, medical, dental and drug prices.

Consumption : An old term applied to pulmonary tuberculosis.

Contact : A person or animal that has been in an association with an infected person or animal or a contaminated environment which might provide an opportunity to acquire the infective agent.

Contagion : Transmission of infections by direct contact.

Contamination : Pollution with infective material.

Contingency Coefficient : A measure of the strength of the relationship between two categorical variables.

Contingency Table : A two- or more-way table that categorizes observations as frequency counts.

Continued Stay Review : The review carried on during a patient's hospitalization to determine the medical necessity of continuation of care at that level.

Continuous Data : Data that can assume any value in a given range.

Continuous Variable : A variable with an infinite number of values.

Contraception : Prevention of conception or impregnation.

Contraceptive Prevalence Rate : The percentage of married women of child-bearing age who are using, or whose husbands are using, any form of contraception, whether modern or traditional.

Contracture : Permanent shortening of muscle.

Control Group : In experimental research, a group that is used as a comparison group to help isolate the influence of an independent variable on a dependent variable.

Controlled Trial : A trial in which subjects are assigned to a control condition as well as to an experimental condition.

Controller : Manager of a hospital's finances; also advises the administrator on financial policy.

Contusion : A bruise.

Convalescence : The period of recovery from an illness.

Convenience Sampling : The selection of a sample that can be obtained simply and conveniently.

Converse Rule : The probability of an event not occurring, equals one minus the probability that it does.

Convulsion : Violent, spasmodic, involuntary muscular movement.

Cornea : The curved, transparent tissue over the iris and pupil on the outside of the eye.

Corns : Horny skin thickenings about the size of peas which occur principally on or between the toes.

Coronary Thrombosis : The occlusion, partial or complete, of a coronary artery by a thrombus (blood clot).

Correlogram : A graph illustrating the autocorrelations between members of a time series (vertical axis) for different separations in time *k* (horizontal axis).

Correlation Coefficient : An index of the degree of association between two variables (ranging from –1 to +1). The higher the absolute value of the correlation coefficient, the stronger the relationship between the two variables.

Correlational Research : Research that does not control and manipulate variables—examines the covariance among variables.

Correlated Samples : A research design in which the scores of one experimental condition are not independent of scores of another experimental condition.

Cost-benefit Analysis : A method of determining and comparing the costs and benefits of a programme in which all the costs and benefits are expressed in monetary terms.

Cost-effectiveness : The relationship between cost and effectiveness, the degree of effectiveness being understood as the extent to which a programme contributes to the attainment of the objectives or improving an unsatisfactory situation.

Cost-effectiveness Analysis : A form of economic evaluation where the costs are expressed in money terms where some of the consequences are expressed in physical units (*e.g.* life-years gained, cases detected).

Cost Efficiency : The relationship between cost and efficiency, the extent to which the resources of a programme are being used as well as possible.

Cost of Uncertainty : The smallest expected opportunity loss in a decision-making problem involving uncertainty.

Cost-utility Analysis : An economic analysis in which outcomes are measured in terms of their social value (*e.g.* "quality adjusted life years" or "healthy days of life").

Counter Balancing : A strategy used with repeated measures designs in which subjects differ by the order in which experimental conditions are presented.

Courtesy Medical Staff : Physicians or dentists who have privileges to admit patients only occasionally.

Covariance : A measure of the tendency of two continuous measurements to vary together.

Co-variation : The tendency of two continuous measurements to vary together.

Covarimin : A criterion for obtaining an oblique rotation; a variation of indirect oblimin rotation.

Coverage : A measure of the extent to which the services rendered cover the potential need for these services in a community.

Cox Regression : A regression method used when the outcome is censored. The regression coefficients are interpreted as adjusted relative risk or odds ratios.

Cramer's Phi : A measure of the strength of the relationship between two variables, both of which are categorical.

Cramp : A painful, spasmodic, involuntary muscular contraction.

Craniotomy : Surgical opening into the skull cavity.

Cranium : The skull; the brain-containing part.

Cretinism : A condition resulting from thyroid deficiency in foetal or early neonatal life, characterized by stunted physical and mental development.

Criteria : Predetermined elements of health care, the presence, absence, and completeness of which indicate the quality of medical services.

Criteria Mapping : System for selecting cases for review from hospital records, using maps outlining a sequence of decisions which should be taken and action which should be initiated during care of specified types of patient.

Criterion : The variable being predicted in a linear regression analysis; a dependent variable.

Criterion Significance : A numerical value or decision rule that specifies when the null hypothesis is to be rejected.

Critical Interval : When computing percentiles, the class interval in which the specified raw score or critical case number falls.

Critical Region : The area under a curve that has the values that lead to rejection of the null hypothesis.

Critical Value : The value that separates the critical region from those values of the test statistic that would not lead to the rejection of the null hypothesis.

Cross Cultural Study : A study in which populations from different cultural backgrounds are compared.

Cross-Over Design : An experimental design in which each subject receives all the treatments under comparison, in a random order, each subject corresponding to a block in a *randomized block design.*

Cross-Sectional Study/Survey : A study in which data are collected at one fixed point in time from respondents by questioning, examination or investigation.

Cross-Tabulation : A frequency and per cent table of two or more variables taken together.

Croup : Difficult, laborious, raspy breathing and barky coughing of a child.

Crude Birth Rate : The total deaths occurring in a given population in a year divided by the corresponding population at mid-year. usually expressed as a rate per 1000 population.

Crude Marriage Rate : Number of marriages per year per 1000 population.

Crude Mortality (or Death) Rate : The total number of deaths in a geographical area during a time period, divided by the estimated population of the area – usually expressed per 1000 persons per year.

Crude Rate : A rate for the entire population that is not specific or adjusted for any given subset of the population.

Crux : A crucial point, the essential or most important point; a critical moment.

Cryogenics : The study and use of devices utilizing properties of materials near absolute zero in temperature.

Cryosurgery : The use of cold; destroying tissue by freezing.

Cryptorchidism : Failure of the testicles to descend into the scrotum during foetal development.

Culture Shock : A state of social isolation, anxiety, and depression arising when an individual is suddenly placed in an alien culture, or reenters his or her own culture after a prolonged absence.

Cumulative Death Rate : The proportion of a group that dies over a specified time interval. It may refer to all deaths or to deaths from specific cause(s).

Cumulative Frequency Distribution : A frequency distribution which includes a column that indicates the total frequency of scores up to and including a given class interval.

Cumulative Frequency Polygon : A graphic method in which cumulative frequencies or cumulative percentages are depicted.

Cumulative Percentage : The per cent of cases having any score or a score that is lower.

Curettage : The scraping of the lining of a cavity with a curette for diagnostic or therapeutic purposes.

Cuspid : A canine tooth.

Cuticle : The horny outer layer of skin.

Curvilinear Correlation : A relationship between X and Y that begins as either positive or negative and then reverses direction.

Cyanosis : The bluish discolouration of the skin and mucous membrane induced by deficient oxygenation of the blood.

Cybernetics : The study of control and communication in man and the machine, characterized by automatic feedback and control.

Cyclic Effect : A periodic movement in a time series that occurs as a result of stimuli from the economy and is generally not predictable.

Cyst : A sac or cavity, with a definite wall.

Cystectomy : Surgical excision of the urinary bladder.

Cystic Fibrosis : An inherited diseases of the exocrine glands which pour secretions into or out of the body rather than into the blood.

Cystic Kidney : A cognetial condition in which the kidneys are filled with bubble like cysts.

Cystitis : Inflammation of the urinary bladder.

Cystocoele : Sagging of the base of the bladder into the vaginal canal.

Cystoscope : An instrument for examining the interior of the urinary bladder.

Cytology : The study of the cell.

Cytoplasm : The substance of a cell outside of its nucleus.

Cytotoxic : Destructive of cells.

D

Daily Calorie Supply per Capita : The calorie equivalent of the net food supplies in a country, divided by the population, per day.

Daily Census, Average : Average number of inpatients present each day for a given period of time.

Dandruff : Fine, whitish, somewhat greasy scales formed upon the skull.

D & C : Dilation and curettage. An operation in which the uterine canal is dilated and the lining of the uterus scraped with an instrument called a curet.

Data : Material serving as a basis for discussion, inference evaluation and decision.

Data Base : A collection of structured data. The structure of the data is independent of any particular application.

Data Collection : The act or process of locating and recording data for use in analysis and evaluation.

Data Processing : Handling of data according to precise rules of procedure to accomplish such operations as classifying, sorting, calculating, summarizing and recording.

Data Transformation : The expression of data in units other than the original units of measurement.

Days of Stay : The sum of the day's stay of any group of inpatients discharged during a specified period of time.

Death Certificate : A vital record signed by a licensed physician that includes cause of death, decedent's name, sex, birth date, and place of residence and death.

Death Rate : An estimate of the proportion of a population that dies during a specified time period.

Debridement : Surgical cleaning of a wound; removal of foreign material and devitalized tissue.

Debt Service : The sum of principal repayments and interest payments on total external debt.

Debug : To detect, identify the source, and fix errors in a computer programme.

Decibel : The unit of measurement of the loudness of sound, used in tests of hearing.

Deciduous Teeth : Baby teeth; the teeth which are shed when the permanent teeth erupt.

Deciles : Percentile ranks which divide the 100-unit scale by tens.

Decision Analysis : The logical and quantitative analysis of all the factors that influence a decision.

Decision Factors : Those factors or variables that can be changed, manipulated or controlled to achieve the desired objective.

Decision Tree : A diagram of a set of possible actions with their probabilities and the values of the outcomes listed; used to analyze a decision process.

Declaration of Helsinki : A statement by the World Health Organization (W.H.O.) that provides ethical guidelines to researchers involved in experiments on human subjects.

Deduction : The use of a hypothesis that has been fitted to observed facts and applying rules of logic to arrive at various consequences.

De Facto : In demography, implying an actual presence (of a person) or occurrence (of an event) within an area.

Defecation : Passage of faeces; evacuation of the bowels.

Deficiency Diseases : Those caused by insufficiency of some constituents of the diet, such as vitamins, minerals, etc.

Definition : An arbitrarily imposed description that allows common understanding.

Deforestation : The permanent clearing of forest lands for shifting cultivation, permanent agriculture, or settlements.

Degrees of Freedom (D.F.) : The number of independent comparisons that can be made between the members of a sample.

Dehydration : Removal of water from the body, or the state produced by such removal.

De Jure : In demography, implying a formal belonging (of a person) to an area by virtue of residence.

Dentures : The set of natural teeth; also a set of artificial teeth; "plates", "false teeth".

Delirium : A state of extreme mental and motor excitement characterized by delusions and restlessness.

Delivery : The act of giving birth to either a living child or to a dead foetus by manual, instrumental, or surgical means.

Delphi Method : A method for forecasting in the absence of a relevant data base in which a sequence of questionnaires is used to identify the factors that can be of assistance in focussing attention on the resultant forecast.

Delta : In power analysis, an index that combines the population effect size and the sample size.

Delusion : A belief that is not in accordance with facts, and cannot be corrected by an appeal to the reason of the person in question.

Demand—Met : A health need, however identified, that has been handled by one of the branches of the health service.

Demand—Stifled : Perceived health need that is not translated into overt demand due to "bottlenecks" in the provision of facilities.

Demand—Unmet : Request for health care that has not been fulfilled at a point of time (*e.g.* waiting lists and other forms of queues for health care).

Dementia : The state of mental degeneration, due to organic causes, characterized by impairment of comprehension and memory, emotional instability, and changes in character.

Demographic Analysis : A group of techniques for estimating basic demographic variables from census or household survey data on the basis of assumptions about the nature of the population being studied.

Demographic Transition : The transition from high to low fertility and mortality rates, usually related to technological change and industrialization.

Demographer : A specialist in the study of human populations—their size, composition, distribution, migration, and vital statistics, as well as the relation of population trends to social and economic developments.

Demography : The empirical, statistical, and mathematical study of human populations.

Dengue : A disease caused by group B arbovirus transmitted by *Aedes aegypti* mosquitoes and characterized by intense pain.

Denominator : The lower portion of a fraction used to calculate a rate or ratio.

Density of Population : Demographic term meaning numbers of persons in relation to available space.

Dental Visits : Visits to a dentist's office for treatment or advice including services by a technician or hygienist acting under the dentist's supervision. Services provided as hospital inpatients are not included.

Dentist : A doctor who treats the teeth and tissues of the mouth.

Dentistry : The study of the teeth and tissues of the mouth.

Deontology: The study of medical ethics.

Dependency Ratio : Proportion of children (under 15) and old people (over 65) in a population in comparison to all others, *i.e.* the proportion of economically inactive to economically active.

Dependent Variable : A variable the value of which is dependent on the effect of other (independent) variable(s), in the relationship under study.

Depilation : Removal of hair.

Depreciation : Decrease in the value of a capital good because of passage of time, wear and tear, etc.

Depression : An emotional state of dejection and unhappiness.

Dermatitis : Inflammation of the skin, often called eczema.

Dermatologist : A specialist in skin problems.

Dermatology : The study of the skin and its diseases.

Descriptive Statistics : Statistics used as the mean, the standard deviation, the proportion, and the rate used to describe attributes of a set of data.

Descriptive Study : A study designed only to describe the existing distribution of variables, without regard to causal or other hypotheses.

Deseasonalized Figures : Original data adjusted for seasonal movements.

Desensitization : The process of removing an individual's sensitivity to a given factor, as in the treatment of allergic conditions.

Design Matrix : A specification, expressed in matrix format, of the particular effects and combinations of effects that are to be considered in an analysis.

Determinant : Any factor that brings about change in a health condition, or other defined characteristic.

Deterministic Model : A model that contains no random elements, as opposed to a probabilistic model.

Detoxification : The process of removing the toxic factors from micro-organisms or poisons.

Deviation : The distance and direction of any raw score from the mean.

Deviation Score (X) : The difference between a single score and the mean of the distribution—found by subtracting the mean $\overline{X}$ from the score X.

Diabetes Mellitus : A metabolic disorder due to lack of insulin, characterized by high blood sugar and usually glycosuria.

Diagnosis : A condition for which a patient needs, seeks, or receives medical care. **Principal Diagnosis** : The condition established after study to be chiefly responsible for occasioning the admission of the patient to the hospital for care. **Other Diagnoses** : All conditions that coexist at the time of admission, that develop subsequently, or that affect the treatment received or length of stay.

Diagnostic Index : A system for recording diagnoses, diseases, or problems of patients in a medical service, usually including identifying information and dates of encounters.

Diagnostic Services : All services that are performed or ordered pertinent to the patient's reasons for the encounter (*e.g.* history, physical examination, laboratory, X-rays, etc.).

Dialysis : Separation of substances in solution by passing them through a porous membrane; this is done mechanically by an artificial kidney.

Diastole : The "resting" stage of the heart during which relaxed chambers are filling with blood.

Diarrhoea : Excessive evacuation of the bowels.

Diathermy : Generation of heat in body tissues by passing high-frequency electric currents through them.

Dichotomous Observation : A nominal measure that has only two outcomes (*e.g.* male or female, yes or no); also called binary.

Dietitian (or Dietician) : A person who is trained in nutrition and plans meals for hospital inpatients.

Diphtheria : An acute infective disease caused by *Corynebacterium diphtheriae,* and characterized by a membranous exudate, usually in the tonsillar region.

Dipsomania : Compulsion to drink alcoholoic beverages to excess.

Direct Obstetric Death : The death of a woman resulting from obstetric complications of the pregnancy state, labour, or puerperium—from intervention, omissions, or treatment, or from a chain of events resulting from any of the above.

Director of Nursing : Nurse responsible for the nursing staff in a hospital.

Disability : Any short-or long-term reduction of a person's activity as a result of an acute or chronic condition; often measured in terms of the number of days by which a person's activity has been reduced.

Disbursement : The release of funds to, or the purchase of goods or services for, a recipient; by extension, the amount thus spent.

Discharge : The termination of a period of inpatient hospitalization through the formal release of the inpatient by the hospital.

Discharge Analysis : The tabulation of data on discharged hospital patients to reflect the professional services provided in the hospital.

Discharge Status (Disposition of Patient) : A record of the condition of the patient on discharge, recommended treatment, and other information necessary for follow-up care.

Discharge Transfer : The disposition of an inpatient to another health care institution at the time of discharge.

Discordant : A term used in matched pair case control studies to describe a pair whose numbers had different exposures to the risk factor under study.

Discrete Data : Data that can be arranged into naturally occurring or arbitrarily selected groups as opposed to data in which there are no naturally occurring breaks in continuity, *i.e.* continuous data.

Discrimination Ratio : The ratio of the specified reliability to minimum acceptable reliability.

Discriminant Analysis : A statistical technique used with discrete dependent variables, concerned with separating sets of observed values and allocating new values.

Disease : A departure from the recognized norms of health. An illness of a specific, defined type, recognizable by its characteristic features.

Disease and Operation Index : A numerical index of patient problems, diagnoses, and procedures by individual categories.

Disease Control : All the measures designed to prevent or reduce the incidence, prevalence, and consequences of disease, such as the control of disease vectors, immunization, curative care, etc.

Disease Prevention : Measures for preventing the occurrence of disease and the arrest of its progress and reduction of its consequences once it is established.

Disease Staging : System for categorizing patients and cases according to severity of illness.

Disease Surveillance : The continuing scrutiny of all aspects of occurrence and spread of diseases to detect changes in trends or distribution, as a basis for integrating control measures.

Disinfection : Killing of infectious agents outside the body by direct exposure to chemical or physical agents.

Disinfestation : Any physical or chemical process serving to destroy or remove undesired small animal forms present upon the person, the clothing or in the environment of an individual, or on domestic animals.

Disjoint Events : Events that cannot occur at the same time.

Disk : A flat circular plate with a magnetizable surface layer on which data can be stored by magnetic recording.

Dislocation : Displacement of a bone from its normal position in a joint, usually the result of a severe blow or fall.

Disorientation : The mental state in which the individual is confused as to place, time and identity.

Dispersion : The spread, or variability, in a set of data.

Displaced Person : Person who is compelled to migrate, usually by a public authority.

Distance Measure : A measure that describes dispersion in terms of the distance between the values of selected observations.

Distribution : The complete summary of the frequencies of the values or categories of a measurement made on a group of persons.

Distribution-Free Test : In inferential statistics, tests that do not make assumptions about characteristics of the population distribution.

Diuretic : A drug that induces diuresis (increased secretion of urine).

Divorce Rate : Number of divorces and legal separations per year per 1000 population.

Divorce Ratio : Number of divorces and legal separations per year per 100 existing marriages or per 100 marriages that year.

DMF : In dental epidemiology, abbreviation used for *d*ecayed, *m*issing, and *f*illed teeth.

DNA (Deoxyribonucleic Acid) : A nucleic acid found in the cell nucleus where it forms part of the fundamental genetic material of the chromosome. It is the carrier of genetic information in living cells.

Doctors : Refers to physicians and includes all graduates of any faculty or school of medicine in any medical field (including practice, teaching, administration and research).

Documentation : Orderly presentation, organization and communication of recorded specialized knowledge, in order to maintain a complete record of reasons for changes in variables.

Dosage Form : The form of the completed pharmaceutical product, *e.g.* tablet, capsule, elixir, suppository.

Dose : The quantity of a given medicament to be given at one time.

Dosimetry : The accurate determination of doses, used particularly in deep X-ray therapy.

Dot Plot : A graphical method for displaying the frequency distribution of numerical observations for one or more groups.

Double Blind Trial : A clinical trial in which neither the subjects nor the investigator(s) know which treatment subjects have received.

Down Time : Total time during which the system is not in acceptable operating condition.

Dressing : A bandage that usually covers the sutures or stitches after a surgical procedure.

DRG (Diagnosis Related Groups) : A system for determining reimbursement based on the admission designation of the patient. The institutions would be reimbursed a set amount, regardless of length of stay.

Drip : The continuous slow introduction of a fluid.

Drives : In computers, that part of the system which is used to read the memory. Generally, three drives are available — called A, B and C. The first two are used to read floppy disks or diskettes and the last refers to the hard disk.

Drug : Any substance in a pharmaceutical product that is used to modify or explore physiological systems or pathological states for the benefit of the recipient.

Drug Formulation : The composition of a dosage form, including the characteristics of its raw materials and the operations required to process it.

Drug Utilization : The marketing, distribution, prescription and use of drugs in a society, with special emphasis on the resulting medical, social and economic consequences.

Dummy Coding : A procedure in which a code of zero or 1 is assigned to a nominal predictor variable used in regression analysis.

Dummy Variable : A qualitative variable included in regression analysis.

Dunnett's Procedure : A multiple-comparison method for comparing multiple treatment groups with a single control group following a significant F-test in analysis of variance.

Durbin-Watson Test : A test for the presence of autocorrelation.

Dwelling : In demography, any inhabited structure such as a house, hut, or tent (with its own entrance and cooking facilities) where one or more households are living.

Dyscrasia : Abnormal state, especially of the blood.

Dysentery : Inflammation of the colon, resulting in the passage of frequent, watery, sometimes bloodstained stools.

Dysfunction : Abnormality or impairment of the normal activity of an organ or bodily process.

Dyslexia : Inability to read efficiently.

Dysmenorrhea : Difficult, painful menstruation.

Dyspareunia : Painful or difficult sexual intercourse; the cause may be physical, psychic, or both.

Dyspepsia : Disturbed digestion; indigestion.

Dyspnea : Difficult or laboured breathing.

Dystocia : Painful or difficult labour, delivery, childbirth.

Dystrophy : Degeneration, wasting, abnormal development.

Dysuria : Difficult or painful urination.

E

Early Foetal Death : Death of a foetus of less than 20 weeks' gestation, 500 grams or less.

Echoviruses : A group of viruses, the name being based on the first letters of their full name : *E*nteric *C*ytopathogenic *H*uman *O*rphan, which are responsible for a range of diseases in man.

ECG (or EKG) : Electrocardiogram. A recording of heart movements on paper through electronic impulses, used in the diagnosis of heart problems.

Eclampsia : The complication of pregnancy characterized by convulsions, proteinuria and hypertension.

E-Code : The ICD-9 Code for the *external* cause of an injury, poisoning, or adverse effect.

Ecology : The study of the relationship among living organisms and their environment.

Ecological Correlation : A correlation in which the units studied are populations rather than individuals.

Ecological Fallacy (or Bias) : The bias that may occur because an association observed between variables on an aggregate level does not necessarily represent the association that exists at an individual level.

Econometric Model : A set of two or more simultaneous mathematical equations that describe the interrelations among variables in a system.

Economy : Minimum expenditure on resources.

Ectomorph : A tall, thin type of body build.

Ectoparasite : A parasite that lives on the surface of its host.

Ectropion : Out-turning of an eyelid, droping away from the eyeball.

Eczema : Inflammation of the skin, with redness and itching.

Edema : Excessive accumulation of watery fluid in body cavities and spaces around cells.

EEG : Electroencephalogram : A recording of brain waves (on paper) through electronic impulses, used in diagnosing brain disease.

Effective Fertility Ratio : Number of children under age 5 per 100 women in childbearing ages.

Effectiveness : The extent to which a specific intervention, procedure or service, when deployed in the field, does what it is intended to do for a defined population.

Efficacy : The extent to which a specific intervention, procedure or service produces a beneficial result under ideal conditions.

Efficiency : The end-results achieved in relation to the effort expended in terms of money, resources, and time.

Effusion : Outpouring of fluid into a body part or tissue.

Ejaculation : Ejection of semen.

Elaboration : The process of controlling a two-variable cross-tabulation for additional variables.

Elective Treatment : Postponable treatment, not immediately urgent.

Element : One of the parts, principles, materials or traits of a system.

Elephantitis : Gross enlargement of a body part due to fluids in tissue spaces under the skin, due to obstruction of lymphatic drainage channels.

E-Mail (Electronic Mail) : A system for transmitting documents and messages among computer terminals by means of computer communication links.

Embolism : The sudden blocking of a blood vessel by an embolus (a foreign body).

Embryo : The developing human being in the uterus through the third month of pregnancy, after which it is known as a foetus.

Emergency : Any condition in which the life of a patient is in immediate danger and where any delay in administering treatment could add to that danger.

Emergency Care Service : A service provided to outpatients to sustain life or prevent critical consequences and that should be performed immediately, usually hospital-based.

Emergency Unit : Special facility in a hospital where ailments are treated 24 hours a day, 7 days a week.

Emetic : A drug or other means which produces vomiting.

Emphysema : Abnormal presence of air in the tissues.

Empirical Criteria : Criteria derived from actual practice.

Empirical Data : Information that has been verified through observations or experimentation.

Empyema : Accumulation of pus in a body cavity, especially in the pleural cavity.

Enabling Factor : An independent variable derived from those characteristics or attributes which tend to facilitate the occurrence of the dependent variable.

Encephalitis : Inflammation of the brain due to viruses or complications of other diseases.

Encephalopathy : An imprecise term referring to any disease of the brain and, in particular, to any chronic degenerative disease.

Encopresis : Involuntary passage of faeces.

Encounter : A face-to-face transaction between a personal health worker and a patient or client.

Endarterectomy : Surgical removal of a clot or plaque from the inner wall of an artery.

Endemic Disease : The constant presence of a disease or infectious agent within a given geographic area or population group.

Endocarditis : Inflammation of the lining of the heart, especially attacking the heart valves.

Endocrinology : The science dealing with endocrine glands and their internal secretions.

Endodontics : A branch of dentistry concerned with disease and treatment of inner structures of the teeth; pulp, root canal filling, etc.

Endogenons : Growing from or inside the system: arising from internal structural or functional causes.

Endomorph : An obese type of body build .

Endoscopy : Visual examination of hollow parts of the body by insertion of a lighted instrument through a natural outlet.

Enteritis : Inflammation of the intestines.

Enterobiasis : Pinworm infection.

Enteroviruses : Viruses, such as polio and ECHO viruses, whose preferred habitat is the intestinal tract.

Enucleation : Removal of the eyeball.

Enumeration : The listing of or dealing with all the feasible alternatives.

Enuresis : The unconscious or involuntary passage of urine.

Environment : The surroundings of a system. Everything outside a system that either affects the operation of the system or is affected by the system.

Eosinophilia : An increase in the number of eosinophils in the blood.

Eosinophils : Certain white blood cells which accept a rose-coloured stain called eosin.

Epidemic : Unusually frequent occurrence of disease in the light of past experience.

Epidemiology : The study of the factors determining the occurrence of disease in populations.

Epididymitis : Inflammation of that part of the semen-conducting duct which lies upon and behind the testicle.

Epilepsy : A sudden, transient recurring disturbance of cerebral function, characterized by convulsions and loss of consciousness.

Epinephrine : The hormone produced by the medulla of the adrenal gland, also known as adrenaline.

Epsilon : In one-way analysis of variance, a measure that estimates the strength of the relationship between the independent and dependent variables in the population.

Episiotomy : An incision in the margin of the vulva to enlarge the area through which the baby's head passes in childbirth, done to minimize injury to the mother.

Episode : Period in which a health problem or illness exists, from its onset to its resolution.

Epistaxis : Bleeding from the nose.

Epizootic : Epidemic diseases in animals.

Eponym : The name of a person applied to a disease, syndrome, or theory.

Equation : An expression of the equality or relationship between two or more factors.

Equimax : A criterion for obtaining an orthogonal rotation, this criterion is a compromise between varimax and quartimax criteria.

Equity : Fairness. In health care the fair distribution of resources for care and lack of discrimination in access to care.

Ergotism : Poisoning with *ergot,* a substance contained in a fungus that grows on rye and other grains.

Error of Estimation : The difference between an estimated value and the true value.

Error-Free Data : Contrived data where the underlying model is presumed known and there is an exact fit between data and model.

Error Mean Square : In analysis of variance, the error sum of squares divided by the error degrees of freedom.

Error Term (Disturbance Term) : The residual portion of a score that cannot be predicted by the independent variable. Also, the distance of a point from the regression line.

Error Variance : The variation among scores due to uncontrolled random factors in the experiment, within group variance.

Eructation : A belch.

Erysipelas : An acute bacterial infection of the skin and underlying tissue.

Erythema : Abnormal redness of the skin.

Erythroblastosis : A disease of neoborn infants associated with incompatible Rh blood factors of mother and child.

Erythrocytes : Red blood cells, elastic discs containing haemoglobin.

Erythropoiesis : The process of red blood cell formation.

Essential Criteria : Research-based criteria that are predictive of specific outcomes.

Essential Drugs : Therapeutic substances that are indispensable for the rational care of the vast majority of diseases in a given population.

Estimation : In statistics, a function for computing estimates of a parameter from observed data.

Estimator : A statistical measure used to estimate a population parameter *e.g.* the sample mean X is the estimator of the population mean.

Estrogen : A general term for female hormones.

Ethnomedicine : Beliefs and practices relating to disease which are the products of indigenous cultural development and are not derived from the conceptual framework of modern medicine.

Etiology (Aetiology) : The study of the causes of disease.

Eunuch : A castrated male; a boy or man whose testicles have been removed.

Euphoria : Feeling of well-being; often implies exaggerated elation.

Eustachian Tube : A tubular passage leading from the middle ear to the throat.

Euthanasia : Putting to death an individual suffering from incurable and/or painful disease.

Evaluation : A process that determines the relevance, effectiveness, and impact of activities in the light of their objectives.

Event : A subset of the outcomes of an experiment. A collection of sample points.

Exanthem(a) : Disease with skin rash.

Exchange Transfusion : Replacement of all of a baby's blood with suitable blood of a donor.

Excipient : Any component of a finished dosage form other than the claimed therapeutic ingredient or ingredients.

Excision : The surgical removal of an organ or part of it, or tissue.

Excreta, Excrement : Waste matter excreted or discharged from the body.

Exfoliation : Peeling or shedding of surface skin in scales or sheets.

Exhaustive Outcomes : Outcomes that account for ("exhaust") the entire sample space.

Exogenous : Originating from or due to causes outside the system.

Exophthalmos : Bulging eyes, a condition characteristic of thyroid disease.

Exotoxin : Toxin (poison) released by a micro-organism into its micro-environment. *e.g.* tetanus toxin produced by the tetanus bacillus.

Expectation of Life (or Life Expectancy) : The average number of years an individual of a given age is expected to live if current mortality rates continue to apply. (See *Life Expectancy*)

Expected Frequencies : In contingency tables, the frequencies observed if the null hypothesis is true.

Expected Value : The probability of an event occurring multiplied by the payoff or worth (value) associated with its occurrence.

Expectorant : A substance that softens or increases bronchial secretions and helps to "bring up" phlegm from the chest.

Experiment : Any operation capable of replication under essentially stable circumstances. A situation involving uncertainty.

Experimental Design : Techniques used in experimental research for creating equivalent groups of subjects.

Experimental Study : A study in which conditions are under the direct control of the investigator.

Expert System : A computer system containing organized knowledge so that it can perform some of the functions of an expert human consultant.

Explicit Criteria : Predetermined elements against which aspects of the quality of care may be compared.

Exploratory Surgery : Surgery that is performed to help confirm a diagnosis, usually not intended to cure the patient.

Exponential Smoothing : A forecasting method that weights together the current actual figures and current forecast figures to obtain new forecast values.

Exposure : A (potential) cause of disease.

Extended Family : Group of related persons living together, often embracing more than two generations.

Extensor : A muscle which straightens or extend a body part.

External Cause : External events and circumstances as the cause of injury, poisoning and other adverse effect.

External Validity : The extent to which experimental findings can be generalized to a population at large.

Extramural Birth : A newborn delivered in a non-sterile environment.

Extrapolate, Extrapolation : To predict the value of a variate outside the range of observations; the resulting prediction.

Extrasystole : A premature beat of the heart.

Extreme Immaturity : Birth weight of less than 1,000 grams and/or a gestation of less than 28 completed weeks.

Extreme Point Alternative : An alternative or solution that completely utilizes one of the resources available.

Extrinsic Incubation Period : In arthropods, time necessary after acquisition of infection for an agent to multiply sufficiently that it can be transmitted by the arthropod.

Exudate : Anything that is exuded, oozed, trickled, or pushed out.

Eye Tooth : A canine tooth.

F

F Distribution : The probability distribution used to test the equality of two estimates of the variance. It is the distribution used with the F test in ANOVA; named in honour of R.A. Fisher who first described this distribution.

F Ratio : The result of an *analysis* of *variance,* a statistical technique which indicates the size of the between-groups mean square relative to the size of the within-groups mean square.

F Tables : Tables that document the critical values used in *analysis of variance* testing.

F Test : The statistical test for comparing two variances, used in ANOVA.

Facelift : An operation to remove wrinkling caused by loose skin and to tighten fatty tissues which tend to sag in the face and neck with advancing years.

Face Presentation : Appearance of the face of the foetus at the outlet of the uterus during delivery, instead of the top of the head, as is normal.

Facsimile : A process of digitizing a page, transmitting the resulting bit stream, and reconstructing the original material.

Factor : A characteristic that is the focus of inquiry in a study; used in *analysis of variance.*

Factor Analysis : An advanced statistical method for analyzing the relationships among a set of items or indicators to determine the factors or dimensions that underline them.

Factor Effect : A difference between population factor means or between population cell means.

Factor Extraction : The initial stage of factor analysis in which the covariance matrix is resolved into a smaller number of underlying factors or components.

Factor Level : Any of the possible forms of a factor.

Factor Loading : A general term referring to a coefficient in a factor pattern or structure matrix.

Factor Score : The estimate for a case on an underlying factor formed from a linear combination of observed variables; a by-product of the factor analysis.

Factorial : The product of a whole number multiplied by all smaller whole numbers.

Factorial ANOVA : The factorial ANOVA analyzes data from an experiment that has two or more independent variables.

Factorial Complexity : A characteristic of an observed variable; the number of common factors with loadings on that variable.

Factorial Design : In ANOVA, a design in which each subject (or object) receives one level of each factor.

Factorial Determination : The overall degree to which variations in observed variables are accounted by the common factors.

Faeces : Contents of a bowel movement; the stool.

Failure to Thrive : Lack of expected normal physiological development in a child, including lack of weight gain, lack of growth, physical retardation, and short stature.

Faint : Syncope. Temporary loss of consciousness.

Fallout : Radioisotopes from nuclear explosions which settle out of the atmosphere.

False Pregnancy : Signs and symptoms of pregnancy occurring without conception (pseudocyesis).

False-Negative : A test result that is negative in a person who has the disease.

False-Positive : A test result that is positive in a person who does not have the disease.

Familial Disease : Disease that exhibits a tendency to familial occurrence either due to genetic transmission or the family's shared experience, including its exposure to a common environment.

Family of Classifications : In disease classification, a set of related classification schemes describing different aspects of health problems.

Family Numbering : A system in which the family is assigned one number and the individual family members are assigned sub-numbers.

Family Planning : The conscious efforts of couples to regulate the number and timing of their children's births.

Family Study : An epidemiologic study of a family or a group of families to determine whether the characteristic clusters specifically in certain families.

Farmer's Lung : A form of allergic disease of the lungs caused by the inhalation of dust from mouldy hay or straw.

Farsightedness : A condition in which light from near objects is focussed behind rather than upon the retina, usually because the eyeball is too short (hyperopia).

Fatality Rate : Number dying from a disease per 100 having the disease.

Feasibility Analysis : The process that examines, identifies, and ranks alternative solutions to a problem by considering such factors as software, hardware, cost analysis, staffing etc.

Feasible Alternative : An alternative or solution that meets all requirements and does not violate any constraints.

Feasibility Study : An evaluation to determine whether a plan is capable of being accomplished successfully.

Febrile : Characterized by fever.

Fecundity : Biological potential for reproduction.

Fee : The payment received by a physician from a patient for medical services.

Feedback : Provision of information on results of performances for use in modifying future performance.

Feeding Disorder of Childhood : Food refusal and extreme faddiness in the presence of an adequate food supply and a reasonably competent care giver, and in the absence of organic disease.

Female-male Gap : A set of national, regional, and other estimates in which all the figures for females are expressed in relation to the corresponding figures for males, which are indexed to equal 100.

Fertility Control : A deliberate effort on the part of individuals, societies, or social groups to regulate the number of offspring.

Fertility Rate : A measure of the number of births during a given year per 1,000 women of childbearing age, usually defined as ages 15 to 44 or 15 to 49.

Festination : The taking of hurried short steps to prevent falling, characteristic of Parkinson's disease.

Fetish : An inanimate object endowed with human or supernatural properties.

Fetishism : The form of perversion in which sexual excitement is aroused by the sight of clothing or the like belonging to the opposite sex.

Fever : A disease in which the body temperature is raised above normal (*i.e.* 98.4°F or 37°C).

Fibrillation : Tremor of a muscle, especially the heart muscle.

Fibroid : Resembling fibrous tissue. A leiomyoma of the uterus.

Fibrosis : Excessive production of fibrous tissue.

Field Experience : A mode of research involving the response of personnel in a field situation or environment to a test situation.

Field Survey : The planned collection of data in "the field", *i.e.* among non-institutionalized persons in the general population.

Field Workers : A general term covering the entire field staff used to collect information on vital events and the base population.

Fifty-Fifty Fallacy : The erroneous belief that events are equally likely when only two events are possible.

Filariasis : Infestation with the filaria worm (a filiform nematode or roundworm).

File : A collection of related records.

Final Diagnosis : The complete set of discharge diagnoses applicable to a single patient experience such as inpatient hospitalization.

Finite Population : A population in which the number of elements is fixed and countable.

First Aid : The emergency treatment administered to tide a patient over until he can be attended to by a qualified practitioner in hospital or elsewhere.

First Intelligence : The initial indication, sometimes in the form of a mere hint, that a vital event has taken place.

First Quartile : The 25th percentile. .

Fiscal Intermediary : An organization acting in an intermediate role for dispersing funds from the central government.

Fishbone Diagram : A graph used in quality control to identify possible problem causes. Also called an Ishikawa diagram after its inventor.

Fisher's Exact Test : A statistical test of the hypothesis of no association between two variables, used to obtain a 2×2 contingency table (with 2 rows and 2 columns); used when the sample size is too small to use the chi-square test.

Fisher's LSD (Least Significant Difference) : A multiple comparison test used to locate the source of significance following a significant F test.

Fisher's Z Transformation : A transformation of the correlation coefficient so that it is normally distributed.

Fissure : A cleft or groove.

Fistula : An abnormal channel leading from some natural cavity to the exterior or from one such cavity to another.

Fitted Values : In regression analysis, the estimated values of the dependent variable given by the regression equation.

Fitness : In health care, a set of attributes that people have or achieve, that relate to their ability to perform physical activity.

Five-number Summary : A procedure for summarizing important numerical characteristics of a set of data : the median, first and third quartiles, and lowest and highest scores.

Five Per cent Level (.05) of Significance : A level of probability at which the null hypothesis is rejected if an obtained sample difference occurs by chance only 5 times or less out of 100.

Fixed Cohort : A cohort in which membership is fixed by being present at some defining event ("zero time").

Fixed Costs : Those elements of cost that do not vary with volume of production.

Flat-Foot : The deformity of the foot characterized by flattening of the normal arch of the foot.

Flatulence : The presence of excessive gas in the stomach.

Flexor : A muscle which bends a limb or part.

Floaters : Cells or strands of tissue which float in the vitreous humour and move with movement of the eyeball, causing shadows on the retina.

Floppy Disk : A flexible magnetic disk enclosed in a protective container.

Flow Chart : A systematic method of recording information in pictorial form, a graphic representation of the major steps of work in progress.

Flukes : Parasitic flatworms which cause infections of the intestines, liver and lungs.

Fluoridation : The procedure of adding salts of fluoride to drinking water as a prophylactic measure against dental caries.

Fluorosis : The condition resulting from the excessive intake of fluorine.

Flutter : Rapid, fluttery, but rhythmic beats of the heart auricles, resembling fibrillation.

Focussed Review : A review of target areas or cases identified through analysis of the data system as questionable in effective utilization of resources.

Foetal Alcohol Syndrome (FAS) : A pattern of retarded growth, both mental and physical, found in some children of mothers whose alcohol consumption during pregnancy can be classified as hazardous.

Foetal Death : Death prior to the complete expulsion from its mother of a product of human conception, irrespective of the duration of pregnancy. **Early Foetal Death,** less than 20 weeks' gestation, 500 grams or less. **Intermediate Foetal Death,** 20 completed weeks' gestation but less than 28 (between 500 – 1000 grams), **Late Foetal Death,** 28 completed weeks' gestation and over 1,001 grams.

Foetal Death Certificate : A vital record registering a foetal death or stillbirth.

Foetal Death Rate : The number of foetal deaths in a year expressed as a proportion of the total number of births (live births plus foetal deaths) in the same year.

Foetal Death Ratio : A measure of foetal wastage, defined as the number of foetal deaths in a year divided by the number of live births in the same year.

Foetus : The unborn child after the third month of pregnancy; before that it is called an embryo.

Folic Acid : A vitamin important for blood formation.

Follow-up Study : A study in which individuals or populations receiving a specified preventive or therapeutic procedure are followed to assess the outcome of the procedure.

Fomites (sing. Fomes) : Articles (drinking glass. handkerchief etc.) that convey infection to others because they have been contaminated by pathogenic organisms.

Fontannel : The "soft spot" on the top of a baby's head.

Food Poisoning : Intestinal infection caused by bacteria or their toxins in foods.

Foot Drop : Dropping of the foot, due to paralysis or injury of muscles or tendons that extend or lift it.

Force of Morbidity : Theoretical measure of the number of new cases that occur per unit of population-time, *e.g.* person-years at risk; also known as Hazard Rate.

Force of Mortality : The hazard rate of the occurrence of death at a point in time; also known as Actuarial Death Rate.

Forecasting : Attempting to define possible courses of future events; may include estimating probabilities associated with each course of events.

Forensic : Relating to courts of law.

Format: The arrangement of a form, or an organization of forms in a permanent file folder which directs the type of entries, the way entries are made, and the future use of those entries.

Fortran : FORmula TRANslation. Any of several specific procedure-oriented programming languages.

Fortuitous Relationship : Relationship that occurs by chance and needs no further explanation.

Fracture : A break, usually in the continuity of bone.

Fragile X Syndrome : A heritable point defect on the human X chromosome (X 27-28) which makes the chromosome highly susceptible to breakage; cause of moderate to severe intellectual impairment.

Framingham Study : A cohort study of heart disease in which residents (sample) of Framingham, Massachusetts (U.S.A.) have been subjects of investigations of risk factors in relation to the occurrence of heart disease since 1949.

Fraternal Twins : Twins of either sex originating from two separate eggs; they are no more closely related genetically than brothers and sisters.

Free-Standing Day Hospital : A private hospital where only minor operations and other procedures, not requiring overnight stay are performed.

Frequency : The number of times a given value of an observation occurs; also called counts.

Frequency Curve : A curve used to obtain probabilities by calculating areas under the curve.

Frequency Distribution : In a set of numerical observations, the list of values that occur along with the frequency of their occurrence; may be set up as a frequency table or as a graph.

Frequency Histogram : A specification of the way in which the frequencies of members of a population are distributed according to the values of the variates they exhibit.

Frequency Polygon : A line graph connecting the midpoints of the tops of the columns of a histogram; useful in comparing two frequency distributions.

Frequency Table : A table showing the number or percentage of observations occurring at different values of a characteristic or variable.

Frigidity : Lack or loss of sexual desire in women.

Frozen Shoulder : Pain, stiffness, and limitation of movement in the shoulder and upper arm.

Friedman Test : A non-parametric test used to compare three or more populations of repeated measurements.

Fumigation : Any process by which the killing of animal forms is accomplished by the use of gaseous agents.

Function : The action for which a person or system is specially fitted, used or responsible : the activity appropriate to the nature of the system.

Functional Analysis : An approach to the solution of a problem in which the problem is broken down into its component functions and analyzed till a solution is found.

Fungicide : A substance that kills fungi.

Fungus, Fungi : Low forms of plant life, including moulds and yeasts, some of which are capable of causing annoying or serious infection.

Furuncle : A small abscess due to infection in a hair follicle or sweat gland, known more widely as a *boil.*

Future Labour Force Replacement Ratio : The population under 15 divided by a third of the population aged 15-59.

G

Gait : The manner of walking.

Galactocele : A milk-containing cyst in the breast.

Galactorrhoea : Excessive or spontaneous secretion of milk.

Gallbladder : The pear-shaped reservoir for the storage and concentration of bile, lying on the under-surface of the right lobe of the liver.

Gallstones : Stones in the gallbladder; they may or may not cause noticeable symptoms.

Gambler's Fallacy : The erroneous belief that the repeated occurrence of an event increases the probability that the opposite event will occur.

Game Theory : A theory used mainly in systems analysis; concerned with the range of possible reactions to a particular strategy; has applications in disease surveillance and control.

Gamma : A synonym for effect size.

Ganglion : A knot like mass of nerve cells.

Gangrene : Mortification (putrefaction and death) of the flesh.

GANTT Chart : A progress management chart that tracks the progress of a project against a predetermined schedule.

Gargle : A solution used for rinsing the throat.

Gas Gangrene : Infection with certain clostridia, notably *Clostridium welchii.*

Gastrectomy : Surgical excision of part of, or the whole of, the stomach.

Gastric : To do with the stomach.

Gastritis : Inflammation of the stomach.

Gastroenteritis : Inflammation of the stomach and intestine.

Gastroscope : An instrument for inspecting the interior of the stomach.

Gastrostomy : The establishment of an artificial opening in the stomach.

Gateway Drug : An illicit or licit drug, use of which is regarded as opening the way to the use of another drug, usually one viewed as more problematic.

Gaussian Distribution : See *Normal Distribution.*

Gauss-Markoy Theorem : Theorem stating that the least-squares estimators of the intercept and the slope in the population regression line are the best linear unbiased estimators.

Gauze : A thin, open-web tissue used for surgical dressings.

Gavage : Feeding of liquid nutrients into the stomach via a tube.

Gehan's Test : A statistical test of the equality of two survival curves.

Gel : A colloid which is firm in consistency but contains much water.

Gender Identity : A conviction of being either male or female, resulting from the combined effects of biological and psychosocial factors.

Genes : Biological basis of heredity; occupy precisely defined locations on chromosomes.

Gene Pool : The total of all genes possessed by reproductive members of a population.

General Fertility Ratio : Number of births per year per 1,000 women of childbearing ages.

General Paresis : A late form of neurosyphilis resulting from lesions in the central nervous system and characterized by fatigue, lethargy and temperamental changes.

Generalization : Application of results obtained from a sample to a specific population.

Generic : Pertaining to a genus or group.

Genetics : The study of heredity.

Genetic Counselling : Application of the principles of medical genetics to the risks of occurrence of heritable disorders, and the provision of guidance to families and individuals as regards the prevention, diagnosis, prognosis, and management of these disorders.

Genetic Drift : Random variation in gene frequency from generation to generation : most often observed in small populations.

Genetic Epidemiology : Study of the aetiology, distribution, and control of disease in groups of relatives, and with inherited causes of disease in populations.

Genital : Relating to the reproductive tract or to reproduction.

Genitalia : The organs of reproduction.

Genito-urinary : Relating to the genital and urinary organs.

Genotype : The genetic constitution of an individual.

Genus : A taxonomic group intermediate between family and species (pl. *genera*).

Geometric Mean : A mean derived by multiplying the *n* individual values in a seris of observations and calculating the *nth* root.

Geometric Progression : A series of ordered numbers is said to be in geometric progression if the proportion between any two adjacent numbers is the same. For example, the series 3, 9, 27, 81, ... is in geometric progression.

Geriatrics : A branch of medicine dealing with diseases of old age.

Gerontology : The study of old age and the ageing process.

Germ : A microbe. An egg, seed or spore.

German Measles : (Rubella). A viral infection producing a pink rash with characteristic symptoms of headache and slight fever.

Germicide : A substance that kills micro-organisms.

Germination : The beginning of growth in an egg, ovum, seed or spore.

Gestation : Pregnancy.

Gestational Age : The gestational age of a foetus is the elapsed time since conception. In practice the duration of gestation is measured from the first day of the last normal menstrual period; expressed in completed days or completed weeks.

Giardiasis : Diarrhoea induced by *Giardia intestinalis.*

Gigabyte : 1024 megabytes, approximately one billion bytes.

Gigantism : The state of abnormal overgrowth induced by excessive secretion of growth hormone.

Gingivitis : Inflammation of the gums.

Glandular Fever : Infectious mononucleosis. An acute, infectious, febrile disease characterized by enlargement of lymph glands.

Glaucoma : A disease of the eye characterized by raised intra-ocular pressure.

Glomerulonephritis : The form of nephritis in which the primary inflammatory change occurs in the glomeruli. A form of Bright's disease.

Glossitis : Inflammation of the tongue.

Gluteal : Relating to the buttocks.

Glycogen : The form in which carbohydrate is stored in the animal body.

Glycosuria : The presence of an abnormal amount of glucose in the urine.

Goal : A general aim towards which to strive *e.g.* to have primary health care available to everybody.

Goitre: An enlargement of the thyroid gland.

Gold Standard : In diagnostic testing, a procedure that always identifies the true conditions — diseased or disease-free — of a patient.

Gompertz Law : Law dealing with age and mortality. Mortality is high during infancy and lowest in childhood. After age 40 mortality increases logarithmically with age.

Gonads : The primary sex glands, ovaries or testes.

Gonorrhoea : The inflammatory disease of the genito-urinary passages caused by *Neisseria gonorrhoea*.

Goodness of Fit : Degree of agreement between an empirically observed distribution and a mathematical or a theoretical distribution.

Goodness of Fit Test : A chi-square test that examines the degree to which observed data coincide with theoretical expectations.

Gout : A disorder characterized by excess of uric acid in the blood, painful joints and systemic disturbances.

Gramian : A symmetrical square matrix with all eigenvalues greater than or equal to zero.

Grand Mal : Major epilepsy. Characterized by loss of consciousness and epileptic fits.

Grand Mean : The mean of all the scores in an experiment.

Grand Median : In the median test, the median of all the cases (all samples combined).

Grand Total : The total number of observations cross-classified in a contingency table.

Granuloma : A tumour composed of granulation tissue.

Graph : A diagram representing the successive changes in the value of a variable quantity or quantities. See also *Abscissa, Ordinate*.

Gravidity : The number of pregnancies (completed or incomplete) experienced by a woman.

Greenhouse-Geisser Epsilon : A number used to reduce the univariate degrees of freedom when the Greenhouse-Geisser adjusted univariate approach is used.

Greenhouse Index : Net emission of major greenhouse gases, with each gas weighted according to its heat-trapping quality and expressed in metric tons of carbon per capita.

Gripe : A sharp pain in the bowels.

Gross Autopsy Rate : The ratio during any given period of time of all inpatient deaths.

Gross Domestic Investment : Outlays on additions to the fixed assets of the economy plus net changes in the level of inventories.

Gross Domestic Product (GDP) : The total output of goods and servies for final use produced by an economy, by both residents and non-residents, regardless of the allocation to domestic and foreign claims.

Gross Migration : Sum of in- and out-migration.

Gross National Product (GNP) : Comprises GDP plus net factor income from abroad, which is the income residents receive from abroad for factor services (labour and capital), less similar payments made to non-residents who contribute to the domestic economy.

Gross Reproduction Rate : The average number of female children a woman would have if she survived to the end of her childbearing age, and if she were subject to a given set of age-specific fertility rates and a given sex-ratio at birth.

Group Practice : Care provided by a group of physicians who usually represent a fairly broad spectrum of medical specialities.

Grouped Frequency Distribution : Scores that are arranged into equal-sized class intervals. The number of scores occurring in each interval is placed in a column adjacent to the appropriate class interval.

Growth Hormone : A pituitary hormone whose deficiency results in dwarfism and excess production leads to gigantism and acromegaly.

Growth Rate of Population : A measure of population growth comprising addition of newborn to the population and subtraction of deaths. (The difference between crude birth rate and crude death rate.)

Guidelines : Steps to be taken in performing a task or implementing a policy and the manner of doing so. Based on guiding Principles.

Guiding Principles : General Rules that can be used as a guide by individuals or institutions to develop and implement policies.

Gumboil : A dental abscess causing swelling of the gums.

Gumma : The granulomatous growth of tertiary syphilis.

Gustatory : Pertaining to the sense of taste.

Gynaecologist : A specialist in diseases peculiar to women.

Gynaecology : The branch of medicine concerned with diseases peculiar to women.

Gynaecomastia : Excessive development of the male breast.

H

Habit Forming : Having characteristics that encourage customary or regular use; said of a drug that has substantial dependence potential.

Habituation : Becoming accustomed to any behaviour or condition, including psychoactive substance use.

Haematemesis : Vomiting of blood.

Haematocoele : A swelling produced by effusion of blood into a cavity.

Haematoma : A swelling filled with blood which clots to form a solid mass.

Haemodialysis : Separation of waste materials from blood by passage through a semipermeable membrane, especially as performed by an artificial kidney.

Haemoptysis : Spitting of blood that originates in the chest.

Haematuria : The presence of blood in the urine.

Haemoglobin : An iron-containing protein present in the red blood cells and responsible for the transmission of oxygen from the lungs to the tissues.

Haemolysis : The release of haemoglobin from the erythrocytes.

Haemophilia : A hereditary disease of males, transmitted by females, characterized by bleeding due to marked prolongation of the coagulation time.

Haemopoiesis : The formation of blood.

Haemorrhage : Bleeding. The escape of blood from a blood vessel.

Haemorrhoidectomy : Surgical excision of haemorrhoids.

Haemorrhoids : Piles. A varicose state of the external haemorrhoidal veins.

Haemostasis : The arrest of bleeding.

Half-life : The period during which the activity of a radioactive substance is reduced to one-half of its original value.

Halfway House : A place of residence that acts as an intermediate stage between an inpatient or residential therapeutic programme and fully independent living in the community.

Halitosis : Offensive breath.

Hallucination : A sensory perception of any modality, occurring in the absence of the appropriate external stimulation.

Hallucinogen : A chemical agent that induces alternations in perception, thinking, and feeling which resemble those of the functional psychoses without producing the gross impairment of memory and orientation characteristic of the organic syndromes.

Halo Effect : The influence upon an observation of the observer's perception of the characteristics of the individual observed, or the influence of the observer's recollection or knowledge of findings on a previous occasion.

Hamstring : One of the tendons bounding the popliteal fossa.

Handicap : Reduction in a person's capacity to fulfil a social role as a consequence of an impairment, inadequate training for the role, or other circumstances.

Hangover : A post-intoxication state comprising the immediate after-effects of drinking alcoholic beverages in excess.

Hard Copy : A printed version of the inputs or outputs.

Hard Disk : A rigid disk with much greater memory capacity than a floppy disk, usually permanently sealed in its drive unit.

Hardware : Physical equipment used in data processing, as opposed to computer programmes, procedures, rules and associated documentation.

Hardy-Weinberg Law : The principle that both gene and genotype frequencies will remain in equilibrium in an infinitely large population in the absence of mutation, migration, selection and non-random mating.

Harelip : A congenital fissure in the upper lip.

Hashish : The resin of *Cannabis sativa,* smoked or chewed for its intoxicating effects.

Hawthorne Effect : The effect (usually positive) of being under study upon the persons being studied; their knowledge of the study often influences their behaviour.

Hay Fever : An allergic condition of the mucous membrane of the nose, eyes, and upper air passages, caused by an allergic reaction to pollen.

Hazard : A factor or exposure that may adversely affect health.

Hazard Function : The probability that a person dies in a certain time interval, given that the person has lived until the beginning of the interval; its reciprocal is *Mean Survival Time.*

Hazard Rate : A theoretical measure of the risk of occurrence of an event, *e.g.*, death, new disease, at a point in time.

Health : The state of being free from disease mentally and physically, and the body functioning in all respects at its optimum level of efficiency.

Health Accounting : System of cost benefit analysis in which quality is determined by balance of benefits of specified treatments or procedures over their costs.

Health Behaviour : The combination of knowledge, practices, and attitudes that together contribute to motivate the actions people take regarding health.

Health Care : All services designed to improve health, well-being, and health related aspects of quality of life.

Health Care Services : Processes that directly or indirectly contribute to the health and well-being of patients, such as medical, dental, nursing, and other health-related services.

Health Centre : A centre that carries out promotive, protective, preventive, diagnostic, curative and rehabilitative activities for ambulant people.

Health Development : The process of continuous, progressive improvement of the health status of a population.

Health Education : The process by which individuals and groups of people learn to promote, maintain or restore health.

Health Expenditure : Expenditure by a government on national health and medical insurance schemes, and on family planning and preventive care.

Health Facility Deaths : Deaths occurring after lodging a patient in an inpaient bed.

Health Index : A numerical indication of the health of a given population derived from a specified composite formula.

Health Indicator : A variable. Susceptible to direct measurement, that reflects the state of health of persons in a community. (*e.g.* Infant Mortality Rates, Incidence and Prevalence Rates of Diseases.)

Health Information : Any data pertaining to the physical, mental, or social well-being of an individual or group of individuals.

Health Maintenance Organization (HMO) : A prepaid health plan delivering comprehensive care to members through designated providers, having a fixed monthly payment for health care services, and requiring members to be in a plan for a specified period of time (usually 1 year).

Health Manpower Development : The planning, production and management of health manpower.

Health Need – Perceived : A need when the individual identifies an "abnormality", and which he/she brings to the attention of the medical profession.

Health Need — Unperceived : A condition that is unrecognised by an individual, but is potentially discoverable by a practitioner on careful investigation of the total physical and mental well-being of the individual.

Health Planning : The process of delineation of health goals, definition of health objectives, and specification of health targets for the formulation, implementation and evaluation of health plans.

Health Policy : A set of statements and decisions defining health policies and main directions for attaining health goals.

Health Promotion : An evolving concept that encompasses fostering life-styles and other social, economic, environmental, and personal factors conducive to health.

Health Protection : Guarding against potential dangers to health, such as taking measures to protect workers against the specific hazards of their work.

Health Record : Documentation of direct or indirect health care services to patients by providers and users of the data in any type of health-related institution.

Health Research : Research on all aspects of health—the factors affecting it, and ways of promoting, protecting and improving it.

Health Resources : All the means available for the operation of a health system, including manpower, buildings, supplies, equipment, funds, knowledge and technology.

Health Risk Appraisal (HRA) : A generic term applied to methods for describing an individual's chances of becoming ill or dying from selected causes.

Health Sector : The sector that includes government ministries and departments, social security and health insurance schemes, voluntary organizations, and private individuals and groups, providing health services.

Health Services : Services that are performed by health care professionals or by others under their direction, for the purpose of promoting, maintaining or restoring health.

Health Services Access : A percentage of the population that can reach appropriate local health services on foot or by local means of transport in no more than one hour.

Health Situation : Health status of a population which also includes measures taken to improve health, the resources being devoted to health, and the degree of people's awareness about their health and ways of improving it.

Health Status : A general term for the state of health of an individual, group or population measured against accepted standards.

Health Status Index : A set of measurements designed to detect short-term fluctuations in the health of members of a population; measurements include physical function, emotional well-being, feelings etc.

Health Statistics : Aggregated data describing and enumerating attributes, events, behaviours, services, resources, outcomes, or costs related to health, disease, and health services.

Health Survey : A survey designed to provide information on the health status of a population; may be descriptive, exploratory, or explanatory.

Health System Infrastructure : The entire structure, including services, facilities, institutions or establishments, organizations, and those operating them for the delivery of a variety of health programmes.

Health Systems Research : Research which focuses on the entire health system. Its objective is to ensure that the system is optimally planned and that programmes are carried out by the health system infrastructure efficiently and with appropriate technology.

Health Team : A group of persons having a common health goal, to the achievement of which each member contributes in accordance with his or her competence and skill and in coordination with the functions of the others.

Health Trends : The present health situation of a population and what led up to it as well as the prospects for the future.

Hearing Aid : An appliance for the amplification of sound to improve the perception of sound by a deaf person.

Heart Attack : Common term for *coronary thrombosis.*

Heartburn : A burning sensation behind the sternum. Pyrosis.

Heatstroke : Heat hyperpyrexia. The condition characterized by a rise of temperature to 106 °F (41 °C) or more, induced by exposure to intense heat.

Helminthiasis : Infestation with parasitic worms.

Hemicrania : Headache limited to one side of the head.

Hemiplegia : Paralysis of one side of the body, usually due to a clot or rupture of a brain artery (stroke).

Hepatitis : Inflammation of the liver. **Infectious Hepatitis :** a disease caused by infection of the liver by a virus spread by faccal contamination.

Hepatomegaly : Enlargement of the liver.

Herbicide : An agent that kills weeds.

Herd Immunity : Resistance of a group to invasion and spread of an infectious agent, based on the immunity of a high proportion of individual members of the group.

Hereditary : Through transmission from ancestors to descendants.

Hermaphroditism : The condition characterized by an individual possessing the gonads of both sexes, with varying degrees of sexual ambiguity.

Hernia : Protrusion of an organ, or part of an organ, through the wall of the cavity in which it lies. **Inguinal Hernia**, a hernia in the inguinal canal. **Hiatus Hernia,** a hernia through the oesophageal hiatus. **Umbilical Hernia**, a hernia through the umbilicus.

Herniorrhaphy : The radical surgical cure for a hernia.

Herpes : A vesicular eruption of the skin, caused by viruses, etc.

Heteroscedasticity : The absence of homogeneity of variance or homoscedasticity.

Heterosexuality : Sexual attraction towards the opposite sex.

Hexose : A monosaccharide containing six carbon atoms in the molecule.

Hierarchical Analysis : An analysis in which inclusion of a higher order interaction term implies the inclusion of all lower order terms.

Hip Bone : A large irregular bone which consists of three parts: the ilium, the ischium, and the pubis. Between them the two hip bones form the pelvic girdle of the lower limbs.

Hirsutism : Excessive growth of hair.

Histamine : An amine, derived from histidine, which is a powerful dilator of capillaries, stimulator of smooth muscles and stimulant of gastric secretions.

Histochemistry : The study of the tissues by means of stains and dyes.

Histogram : A graphical representation of a frequency distribution by means of rectangles whose widths represent the class intervals and whose heights represent the corresponding frequencies.

Histology : The study of the minute structure of the tissues.

Histopathology : The study of the minute structure of pathological tissue.

Histoplasmosis : Systemic infection due to inhalation of dusts containing spores of a species of fungi.

HIstorical Analogy : A method for forecasting the sales of a newly introduced product (or service) that uses the sales history of some previously introduced product as a guide.

Historical Cohort Study : A cohort study that uses existing records or historical data to determine the effect of a risk factor or exposure on a group of patients.

Historical Controls : In clinical trials, previously collected observations on patients used as the control value against which the treatment is compared.

Histotoxic : Poisonous to the tissues.

Hives : See *Urticaria.*

Hodgkin's Disease : Malignancy of the lymph nodes.

Hogben Number : A unique personal identifying number constructed by using a sequence of digits for birthdate, sex, birthplace, and other identifiers; suggested by the English mathematician Lancelot Hogben.

Holendemic Disease : A disease for which a high prevalent level of infection begins early in life and affects most of the child population, leading to a state of equilibrium such that the adult population shows evidence of the disease much less commonly than do the children.

Holistic Approach : The approach utilized in anthropology that integrates a wide variety of disciplines in the study of human behaviour.

Home Care Programme : A programme through which a blend of health and social services is provided to individuals and families in their places of residence to restore health.

Homeostasis : The state of equilibrium in which the body is normally maintained.

Homicides : Includes intentional deaths, non-intentional deaths, and manslaughter but excludes traffic accidents resulting in deaths.

Homoeopathy : The system of therapeutics based on the belief that like cures like (*similia similibus curentur*) and involving the use of very small doses of drugs.

Homoscedasticity (Homogeneity of Variance) : A situation in which the variance on a dependent variable is the same (homogenous) across all levels of the independent variables.

Homosexual : Pertaining to the same sex. An individual who is sexually attracted to the same sex.

Hookworm : The name given to two genera of nematodes or roundworms : Ancylostoma and Necator.

Hordeolum : A stye.

Hormone : A chemical substance which, produced in one part of the body, enters the circulation and is carried to distant organs and tissues to modify their structure and function,

Hormonopoiesis : The production of hormones.

Hormonotherapy : Treatment by the use of hormones; endocrinotherapy.

Hospice Care : A programme of palliative and supportive care services providing physical, psychological, social, and spiritual care for dying persons, their families, and other loved ones.

Hospital : An institution or building intended for receiving the sick and injured, and in which they can receive the appropriate treatment.

Hospitalization : A period in a person's life during which he or she is an inpatient in a single hospital without interruption except by possible intervening leaves of absence.

Hospital-Acquired Infection : See *Nosocomial Infection.*

Hospital Administrator : The chief executive officer of a hospital. He is responsible for seeing that all the services required by the hospital are provided and ensuring that the hospital is run efficiently.

Hospital Ambulatory Care : All hospital-directed preventive, therapeutic, and rehabilitative services provided by physicians and other health care personnel to patients who are not hospital inpatients.

Hospital Autopsy : Post-mortem examination performed by a hospital pathologist on the body of a person who has at some time been a hospital patient.

Hospital Autopsy Rate (adjusted) : The proportion of deaths of hospital patients following which the bodies of the deceased persons are available for autopsy and hospital autopsies are performed.

Hospital Beds : Accommodations with supporting services (such as food, and housekeeping) for hospital inpatients.

Hospital Boards : The policy-making body for the hospital; also known as the *Board of Directors* or *Board of Trustees*.

Hospital Boarder : An individual who receives lodging in the hospital but who is not a hospital patient (*e.g.* parents of a sick child).

Hospital Caesarean Section Rate : The ratio of caesarean sections to deliveries performed in a hospital.

Hospital Death Rate : The proportion of inpatient hospitalizations that end in death, usually expressed as a percentage.

Hospital Discharge Abstract System : Abstraction of a minimum data set from hospital charts for the purpose of producing summary statistics about hospitalized patients.

Hospital Discharge Rate : The number of discharges from hospital during a time period, divided by the estimated mid-year population for the hospital's catchment area; usually expressed per 1,000 persons per year.

Hospital Inpatient : A hospital patient who is provided with room, board, and continuous general nursing service in an area of the hospital where patients generally stay at least overnight.

Hospital Inpatient Autopsy : Post-mortem examination performed by a hospital pathologist on the body of a patient who died during inpatient hospitalization.

Hospital Insurance : A form of protection against unprotected high medical costs.

Hospital Newborn Bassinets : Accommodations with supporting services (such as food and housekeeping) for hospital newborn inpatients : includes bassinets, incubators, and isolettes in the newborn nursery.

Hospital Newborn Inpatient : A hospital patient born in the hospital at the beginning of the current inpatient hospitalization.

Hospital Number : A unique institutional number given to a hospital inpatient to allow for tracking and linkage of multiple records within a data collection system.

Hospital Outpatient Care Unit : An organized unit of a hospital, with facilities and medical services exclusively for patients who are ambulatory and who do not currently require or are not currently receiving services as an inpatient of the hospital.

Hospital Record : A written account of all the services provided the patient from the time of admission until discharge.

Hospital Separation : In hospital statistics, the departure of a patient from hospital without distinguishing whether the patient departed alive or dead.

Host : A person or other living animal, including birds and arthropods, that affords subsistence or lodgment to an infectious agent under natural conditions.

Hostel : Establishment providing board, lodging or accommodation for the aged, disabled, or distressed who cannot live independently but do not need nursing care in a hospital or nursing home.

Household : One or more persons who occupy a dwelling, *i.e.* a place that provides shelter, cooking, washing, and sleeping facilities; may or may not be a family.

Household Sample Survey : A survey of persons in a sample of households, conducted through interview, or by the medium of telephone or questionnaire.

Human Blood Index : Proportion of insect vectors found to contain human blood.

Human Capital : The skills and capabilities generated by investments in education and health.

Human Engineering : That area of human factors which applies scientific knowledge to the design of items to achieve effective man-machine integration and utilization.

Human Immunodeficieney Virus (HIV) : The pathogenic organisms responsible for the acquired immunodeficiency syndrome (AIDS).

Hybrid : The offspring of parents of different species.

Hydatid Disease : Infestation with animal tapeworms which produce clusters of fluid-filled cysts in the lungs and other organs.

Hydrocele : An encysted collection of fluid in the tunica vaginalis testis.

Hydrocephalus : The condition characterized by abnormal accumulation of cerebrospinal fluid within the skull.

Hydrolysis : The chemical process whereby a compound reacts with water, with the production of two or more simpler molecules with the hydroxyl atom in one and the hydrogen atom in another.

Hydrophobia : A common word for *rabies.* The literal meaning of the word is "fear of water".

Hydrostatic : Pertaining to a liquid in equilibrium.

Hydrotherapy : The use of water as a therapeutic measure : *e.g.* as baths, douches and the like.

Hygiene : The science of health.

Hygroscopic : Capable of absorbing moisture.

Hymen : The thin fold of mucous membrane situated at the orifice of the vagina.

Hymenorrhaphy : Surgical suturing of the hymen.

Hypnosis : A state of trance in which the individual becomes responsive to the hypnotist's influence.

Hypnotherapy : The use of hypnotism in therapy.

Hypnotic : Inducing sleep. A substance or procedure that induces sleep.

Hyperacidity : An abnormal degree of acidity.

Hyperemesis Gravidarum : Vomiting of pregnancy, more severe than simple "morning sickness" which may require hospitalization.

Hyperendemic Disease : A disease that is constantly present at a high incidence and/or prevalence rate and affects all age groups equally.

Hypergeometric Distribution : A probability distribution appropriate sampling without replacement.

Hyperhydrosis : Excessive sweating.

Hyperopia : Farsightedness.

Hyperplasia : Abnormal increase in the number of cells in a given tissue or organ.

Hyperpyrexia : Excessively high body temperature : *e.g.* over 106 °F (41 °C).

Hypersecretion : Secretion in excess of the normal.

Hypertension : Abnormally high tension, applied particularly to raised blood pressure.

Hyperthyroidism : (Thyrotoxicosis, Toxic goiter). Overactivity of the thyroid gland.

Hypertrophy : Increase in size of an organ because of overgrowth of cells, without an increase in the number of cells.

Hyperventilation : Increased pulmonary ventilation.

Hypochondriac : A person who is obsessed by excessive introspection about his health, with resultant exaggeration of any minor manifestation of bodily malfunctioning.

Hypodermic : Subcutaneous. Underneath the skin.

Hypoglycaemia : An abnormally low blood giucose concentration which occurs in insulinoma, glycogen storage disease, alcoholism, and liver disease; it may also be a result of hyperinsulinism induced by therapeutic insulin.

Hypokinesia : Diminished power of motor function.

Hypophysis : The pituitary gland.

Hypotension : Abnormally low blood pressure.

Hypothermia : Low temperature, whether induced by disease or exposure, or induced artificially for therapeutic or surgical purposes.

Hypothesis : An idea about the nature of reality which is testable by means of systematic research.

Hypothesis-testing Procedure : A decision rule that specifies the values of a sample statistic for which the null hypothesis will be retained or rejected.

Hypothyroidism : Deficiency of thyroid hormone, leading to a slowing down of mental and physical processes.

Hypoxia : Diminution in the amount of oxygen in the body.

Hysterectomy : Surgical removal of the uterus.

Hysteria : A chronic psychoneurosis characterized by exaggerated histrionic behaviour with a variety of motor and sensory disturbances.

I

Iatrogenic : Resulting from the activity of physicians; said of any adverse condition in a patient resulting from treatment by a physician or surgeon.

I.C.D. : *International Classification of Diseases.* A taxonomical scheme developed by WHO to classify diseases for the purpose of local and international comparison.

ICHPPC : *International Classification of Health Problems in Primary Care*; method of classification for use by physicians in general and family practice throughout the world.

ICIDH : *International Classification of Impairments, Disabilities, and Handicaps.* A WHO effort towards a systematic taxonomy of the consequences of injury and disease.

I.C.P.M. : *International Classification of Procedures in Medicine.* A WHO produced taxonomical scheme for classifying all medical procedures (such as surgical, radiological, laboratory, diagnostic, preventive, etc.) employed in health care.

Icteric : Pertaining to jaundice.

Ideal Research Design : A design for research without reference to the availability of data or feasibility of their collection.

Identical Twins : Twins, always of the same sex and having the same heredity, developing from a single fertilized egg.

Idiocy : Profound degree of mental defect.

Idiopathic : Of unknown origin; usually applied to a disease of unknown origin.

Idiosyncrasy : An individual characteristic. In medicine, it means an abnormal reaction following the administration of a medication.

Ileitis : Inflammation of the ileum.

Illicit Drug : A psychoactive substance, the production, sale, or use of which is prohibited.

Illness Behaviour : Behaviour of persons in response to abnormal body signals. Such behaviour influences the manner in which a person defines his symptoms, takes remedial action, and uses the health care system.

Illusion : A false interpretation of a sensory perception.

Image Factoring : A method of obtaining initial factors; the observed variation is decomposed into (partial) images and anti-images, instead of into common parts and unique parts.

Imbecility : A lesser degree of severe mental abnormality than idiocy.

Immunity : The state of being immune, or of being protected against infection.

Immunity—Acquired : Immunity acquired by the host to a natural pathogen for the host.

Immunity—Active : Immunity developed in response to stimulus by an antigen (infecting agent or vaccine) and usually characterized by presence of antibody produced by the host himself.

Immunity—Natural : Species-determined inherent resistance to a disease agent.

Immunity—Passive : That immunity conferred by anti-body produced in another host and acquired naturally by an infant from its mother, or artificially by administration of an anti-body-containing preparation.

Immunity—Specific : A state of altered responsiveness to a specific substance acquired through immunization or natural infection.

Immunization : The process of inducing immunity.

Immunized : The average vaccination of children under one year of age for the antigens used in the Universal Child Immunization (UCI) programme.

Immunochemistry : That branch of chemistry concerned with the substances participating in the immune process.

Immunoglobulin : Substances in the blood and in certain body fluids other than blood which build immunities to various diseases; loosely synonymous with *antibodies*.

Immunologic Tolerance : State of selective inability to respond immunologically to a specific antigen.

Immunology : The study of immunity and the immune process.

Impacted : Firmly lodged, wedged in place; as in impacted wisdom tooth, embedded in the jawbone.

Impairment : Any loss or abnormality of pyshcological, physiological, or anatomical structure or function.

Implicit Criteria : Subjective, internal opinions that evaluators use in defining good practice; the evaluators must be peer professionals.

Impotence : Inability to perform the sexual act.

Inapparent Infection : The presence of infection in a host without recognizable clinical signs or symptoms; identifiable only by laboratory means. Synonyms : *Asymptomatic, sub-clinical, occult infection.*

Inborn : Innate. Implanted before birth.

Inbreeding : Mating by close relatives.

Inception Rate—Spells : The number of spells of sickness that start during a defined period, divided by the average number of persons exposed to risk during that period.

Incidence : Number of new cases of a disease within a specified period of time.

Incidence Density : The person-time incidence rate; sometimes used to describe the hazard rate.

Incidence-Density Ratio (IDR) : The ratio of two incidence densities.

Incidence Rate : The number of new cases of a disease per year, per 1,000 or 100,000 population.

Incidental Procedure : An integral part of a medical visit which is usually associated with professional services.

Incision : A cut or wound made by a sharp instrument such as a knife or scalpel.

Incompatibility : The state of being incompatible, or unable to exist together, as in the case of blood groups.

Incontinence : Lack of control, whether of the excretion of faeces or urine, the sexual or any other impulse.

Incubation Period : The time interval between invasion by an infectious agent and appearance of the first sign or symptom of the disease in question.

Incubator : A chamber with controlled temperature and humidity for the growth of cells or micro-organisms, or for the treatment of premature infants.

Independence : Two variables are said to be dependent if the distribution of values of one is the same for all values of the other. Two events are said to be independent if the occurrence of one is in no way predictable from the occurrence of the other.

Independent Events : Events that are unrelated. The occurrence of one event does not affect the occurrence of another event.

Independent Observations : Observations such that the random variables representing the first, second, third, ..., and *n*th observations are all independent.

Independent Populations : Populations such that all the observations in any population are independent of all the observations in any of the other populations.

Independent Sample Design : An experimental design in which the scores of one experimental condition are unrelated to (independent of) the scores in any other experimental condition.

Independent Samples Test : A significance test used to compare the sample means of two samples.

Independent Variable : The characteristic being observed or measured that is hypothesized to influence an event or manifestation (the dependent variable) within the defined area of relationships under study : In an experimental design, the treatment variable; in regression, the predictor variable.

Index : An organized, condensed list of data that reflects more extensive data pertaining to one subject or source of information (*e.g.* health status index).

Index Case : The first case in a family or other defined group to come to the attention of the investigator.

Index Group (or Index Series) : In an experiment, the group receiving the experimental regimen; in a case control study, the cases.

Index Number : A summary measure that presents a relative comparison between groups of related items.

Indicators, Performance Indicator : Variables that help to measure changes in a programme directly or indirectly and to assess the extent to which the objectives and targets of a programme are being attained. **Performance Indicator** is a related term which has currency in management analysis of health service delivery.

Indicator Variable : A variable that takes only the values 0 and 1, indicating either the absence or presence of a condition.

Indigestion : Disturbance of the normal process of digestion.

Indirect Obstetric Death : The death of a woman resulting from a previously existing disease, or disease that developed during pregnancy, labour, or the puerperium that was not due to obstetric causes although the physiological effects of pregnancy were partially responsible for the death.

Indirect Patient Data : Information which comes from the patient but requires an interpretation before it is usable.

Individual Plan of Care : Document established to view the patient from the aspect of each health care provider. It pulls all portions of the available information together to develop a coordinated, individual plan for use by health care providers or family in further treatment programmes.

Induced Abortion (or Termination of Pregnancy) : The deliberate removal of a child from the mother's womb, illegal in many countries except when proven need exists to protect the life of the mother.

Induced Abortion Rate : The ratio of induced abortions in a specified period divided by the total number of live births in this specified period, multiplied by 100.

Induction : The process of drawing inferences about a whole set from observations on a few of its members.

Induction Period : The period required for a specific cause to produce disease, the interval from the causal action of a factor to the initiation of the disease.

Inductive Fallacy : An error in logic resulting from over generalizing on the basis of too few observations.

Industrial Hygiene : The discipline that anticipates and controls unhealthy conditions of work to prevent illness among employees.

Infant : A young child. Medically, a child under the age of 1 year. Legally, a minor or someone under the legal age of consent.

Infant Death : Death of a live born infant at any time from the moment of birth to the end of the first year of life.

Infant Mortality Rate : The number of infants (children under the age of one year) who die during a stated year per 1,000 live births occurring in the same year.

Infanticide : The murder of an infant.

Infarct : An area , usually wedge-shaped, of necrotic tissue produced by occlusion of an end-artery.

Infected Individual : A person that harbours an infectious agent and who has either manifest disease or inapparent infection (See *Carrier*).

Infection : Lodgment and multiplication of a microbial agent in the body of man or animal.

Infection Committee : Committee responsible for substantiation of hospital *vs.* non-hospital acquired infections, control of infection, and coordination of all other activities regarding infection control within a hospital.

Infectious Diseases : Diseases transmitted by infections.

Infectivity : 1. Ability of an agent to infect. 2. The proportion of exposures that results in infection.

Infecundity : Sterility or barrenness in women.

Inference : The making of statements, or the process of drawing judgements, about a population on the basis of samples.

Inferential Statistics : The procedure using sample data to make inferences about characteristics of a population.

Infertility : Diminution or absence of ability to produce offspring.

Infestation : Parasitic attack or subsistence on the skin or its appendages, as by insects, mites, or ticks; also used to denote parasitic invasion of the organs and tissues, as by helminths.

Infinite Population : A population in which the number of items is uncountable.

Infirmary : A hospital or place where the sick or infirm are maintained or treated.

Inflammation (Inflammatory Process) : Normal tissue response to cellular injury, characterized by dilation of small blood vessels and mobilization of defence cells.

Influenza : An acute viral infection of the respiratory tract, occurring in isolated cases, epidemics, and pandemics.

Informatics : A comprehensive term to describe all aspects of the development and operation of information systems and the supporting computer methodology and technology.

Information : Knowledge or intelligence; facts, data.

Information Activity List : Any detailed record that provides information about the usage of patient information, *i.e.*, how often it is requested.

Information Centre : An organizational entity charged with providing general support services to informatics users.

Information Retrieval : The study of methods and procedures for recovering specific information from stored data.

Information Support : The supply to and from all concerned, and the constant use of relevant, sensitive and consistent information required for formulating, programming, budgeting, implementing, monitoring, and evaluating the functioning of a programme.

Information System : A system for the collection, storage, processing, and dissemination of information to the users, which may or may not be computerized.

Informed Consent : Voluntary consent given by a subject for participation in an investigation or treatment regimen, after being informed of the purpose, methods, procedures, benefits, and risks.

Inguinal : Pertaining to the groin.

Inhalant : A substance that is or may be taken into the body by way of the nose and trachea (through the respiratory system).

Inheritance : The acquisition of characters or qualities by transmission from parent to offspring.

Injection : The forcing of a liquid into a part, as into the subcutaneous tissues, the blood vessels, or an organ.

Injury : A bodily lesion at organic level resulting from acute exposure to energy (mechanical, thermal, electrical, chemical, etc.) interacting with the body in amounts or rates that exceed the threshold of physiological tolerance.

Injury Control : Includes efforts to both prevent injuries and to minimize the consequences of injury damage.

Injury Prevention : Efforts to prevent agents from reaching people in amounts or at rates that exceed human injury tolerance.

In-migration (Immigration) : Entry into a politico-geographic unit (called immigration if the unit involved is a country).

Inoculation : Introduction of micro-organisms, infective material, serum, or other substances into tissues of living organisms, or culture media.

Inpatient : A patient occupying a bed in a health care institution for the purposes of receiving medical or paramedical treatment.

Inpatient Admission : The formal acceptance by a hospital of a patient who is to be provided with room, board, and continuous nursing service in an area of the hospital where patients generally stay at least overnight.

Inpatient Bed Count : The designated number of available hospital inpatient beds, both occupied and vacant, on any given day.

Inpatient Bed Occupancy Ratio : The proportion of inpatient beds occupied, defined as the ratio of inpatient service days to the inpatient bed count days in the period under consideration; *percent occupancy, occupancy percent, occupation ratio, percentage of occupancy* are other synonymous terms.

Inpatient Census : The number of inpatients present at any one time.

Inpatient Days of Stay (Length of Stay) : The number of calendar days from admission to discharge.

Inpatient Discharge : The termination of a period of inpatient hospitalization through the formal release of the inpatient by the hospital.

Inpatient Service Day : A unit of measure denoting the services received by one inpatient in one 24-hour period. Synonyms : *Inpatient Day, Patient Day.*

Input : Data or similar information needed to perform calculations or analyses.

Input-Output Device : Any user equipment which introduces data into or extracts data from a data communications system.

Insanity : A legal term for mental illness, roughly equivalent to psychosis and implying inability to be responsible for one's acts.

In-Scope : A term used to describe reports of vital events that are properly recorded by some data collection procedure with respect to the fact, time, and place of occurrence. See also *Out-of-Scope.*

Insecticide : Any chemical substance used for the destruction of insects, whether applied as powder, liquid, aerosol, or as a "paint" spray.

Insemination : Introduction of semen into the vagina, by natural means or by artificial insemination.

In situ : In its normal place, confined to the site of origin.

Insomnia : Inability to sleep, abnormal wakefulness.

Inspiration : Inhaling, breathing in.

Inspissated : Thickened, from absorption or evaporation of fluid.

Institutional Population : Persons living under arrangements that exclude them from membership in ordinary family households includes inhabitants of hospitals, prisons, military establishments, boarding schools, hotels, old people's homes, etc.

Instrumental Error : Error due to faults arising in any or in all aspects of a measuring instrument, *i.e.*, calibration, accuracy, precision, and the like.

Insufflation : Blowing gas or powder into a body cavity, as the lungs or vagina.

Insulin : A protein hormone secreted by the pancreas into the blood, where it regulates carbohydrate, lipid, and amino acid metabolism.

Insulin Coma : The deepest level of insulin-induced hypoglycaemia.

Integrated Circuit : A solid state microcircuit consisting of inter-connected semiconductor elements diffused into a single device.

Integument : The skin.

Intensive Care : Nursing care provided to seriously ill patients during which constant attention is paid to the patient's condition.

Intensive Care Unit : A hospital patient care unit for patients with life-threatening conditions who require intensive treatment and continuous monitoring.

Intentional Injury : Injury resulting from deliberate violence inflicted by oneself or another person (*e.g.* assault, suicide, rape, etc.)

Intentional Self-harm : Purposely self-inflicted poisoning or injury. Includes such cases whether or not there is evidence that the person intended to kill himself or herself.

Interaction, Biological Interaction : The effect of system variables on each other. Biological interaction means the interdependent operation of two or more causes to produce, prevent, or control disease.

Intercensal Period : Time between two censuses; usually 10 years for national population censuses.

Intercept : In a regression equation, the predicted value of Y when X is equal to zero.

Interdecile Range : Those scores that include the middlemost 80% of a distribution, or the difference between the first and ninth decile.

Interface : The boundary between two hardware or software systems across which data is transferred.

Interference Phenomenon : State of temporary resistance to infections with other viruses, induced by an existing virus infection : mediated in part by interferon.

Interferon : Protein produced by cells infected with viruses which has the property of blocking viral infection of new cells and suppressing viral multiplication in cells already infected.

Interim Patient Record : A paper record made up primarily of computer printouts in those settings where patient information is maintained on the computer until discharge or cessation of treatment.

Intermediate Care Facility : A facility that provides health-related services to persons with a variety of physical or emotional conditions who do not require the degree of care provided by a hospital or skilled nursing facility but who require the care and services available through institutional facilities.

Intermediate Variable : A variable that occurs in a causal pathway from an independent to a dependent variable.

Intermittent Claudication : Pain in the calf muscles and limping, occurring while walking, due to inadequate blood supply.

Internal Validity : The degree to which an experiment can allow the investigator to make a cause-and-effect statement of the relation between the independent and dependent variable.

Intern : A student doctor who has just received his medical degree and who must work in various hospital departments for a prescribed period of time before getting his/her licence to practice.

Internal Consistency (Reliability) : The degree to which the items on an instrument or test are related to each other and provide a measure of a single characteristic.

Internal Migration : Movement between two politico-geographic areas totally within one country.

Internist : A specialist in internal medicine.

Internship : The position or term of service of an intern in a hospital.

Interpolation : 1. The determination of intermediate values in a series on the basis of observed values. 2. Surgical implementation of tissue.

Interquartile Range (IQR) : The difference between the first and third quartiles.

Interrater Reliability : The reliability between measurements made by two different persons (or raters).

Intersectoral Action : Involvement of government sectors other than the health sector in actions affecting health.

Intersex : An individual who exhibits sexual characteristics of both sexes.

Interval Data : Data that can be ordered and used to compute meaningful distances but lack a non-arbitrary zero point.

Interval Endpoints : The first and last numbers in an interval.

Interval Estimate : An estimate that specifies a range of values.

Interval Scale : A scale of measurement in which equal differences between numbers correspond to equal differences in that which is being measured.

Interval Size : The number of scores in each class interval in a grouped frequency distribution.

Intervening Variable : A variable which is postulated to be a predictor of one or more independent variables.

Intervention : 1. The manoeuvre used in an experimental study; may be a drug or a procedure. 2. Peer review criteria that are applied during the process of medical care of an individual patient which may directly influence the action of the attending physicians during care.

Intervention Study : An epidemiologic investigation designed to test a hypothesized cause-effect relationship by modifying a supposed causal factor in a population.

Intervertebral Disks : Cartilaginous cushions between vertebrae.

Interview Schedule : The precisely designed set of questions used in an interview.

Intoxication : A transient condition following the intake of drugs or alcohol resulting in changes in patterns of physiological, or behavioural functions and responses.

Intradermal : Into or within the skin.

Intramuscular : Into or within a muslcle.

Intrarater Reliability : The reliability between measurements made by the same person (or rater) at two different points in time.

Intrauterine Device (IUD) : A contraceptive device positioned within the uterus for contraceptive purposes.

Intravenous : Into or within a vein; as, "intravenous feedings".

Intrinsic Life Table Birth Rate : Births per 1,000 population per year that would occur given age-specific birth rates and life table age-sex distribution.

Intrinsic Life Table Death Rate : 1,000 times reciprocal of expectation of life at birth as computed from a life table.

Intubation : The insertion of a tube as into the larynx.

Intussusception : Sliding of a part of intestine into its hollow interior; "telescoping", like the pushed-in finger of a glove.

In vitro : Within a glass; observable in a test tube; in an artificial environment.

In vivo : Within the living body.

Iodination : The addition of iodine in a compound (*e.g.* iodized salt).

I.Q. : Intelligence quotient. A number or score derived from performance in an intelligence test which expresses individual success on that test relative to the performance of a normative group on the same test.

Iridectomy : Excision of part of the iris.

Irradiation : Exposure to radiant energy (heat, light, X-rays etc.) for therapeutic or diagnostic purposes.

Irreducible : Incapable of being put back in normal position; said of a hernia.

Irregular Movements : Short, erratic fluctuations in time series that have no discernable pattern.

Irrigation : Washing out of a cavity.

Irritable Bowel Syndrome : Hyperirritability and altered motility of the gastro-intestinal tract present in anxious personalities or following life stress or strain.

Ischaemia : Deficiency of blood in a part, due to functional constriction or actual obstruction of a blood vessel.

Island Population : A group of individuals that is immunologically isolated from larger groups and is unduly susceptible to infection with alien pathogens.

I.S.O. : Abbreviation for *I*nternational *O*rganization for *S*tandardization; a worldwide federation of national standards bodies (ISO member bodies).

Isolate : A segment of the population that is set apart from the rest, by geography, religion, economics, etc. and in which matings take place exclusively with other members of the same population.

Isolation : Separation, for the period of communicability, of infected persons from others in such places and under such conditions so as to prevent or limit the transmission of the infectious agent from those infected to those who are susceptible or who may spread the agent to others.

Isometric : Maintaining, or pertaining to, the same measure of length; of equal dimensions.

Itching : Pruritis; an unpleasant cutaneous sensation, provoking the desire to scratch or rub the skin.

Iterative : Describing a procedure which repeatedly executes a series of operations until some condition is satisfied.

I.V. : Abbreviation for *intravenous*. When a fluid is administered to a patient by means of a small tube or catheter directly into a vein, it is called an I.V.

J

Jacksonian Epilepsy : Convulsions beginning with one local movement, usually with a local brain lesion.

Jacob's Syndrome : Scrotal dermatitis, angular stomatitis and conjunctivitis due to riboflavin deficiency.

Jactitation : Extreme restlessness; tossing about in bed.

Japanese Encephalitis : A virus-caused infection, occurring in eastern Asia, transmitted by the bites of mosquitoes.

Jaundice : A yellowish discoloration of the skin and mucous membranes, due to hyperbilirubinaemia.

JCAH : *Joint Commission for the Accreditation of Hospitals.* Now known as the *Joint Commission for the Accreditation of Health Care Organizations* (JCAHO); US organization which grants accreditation to hospitals and other health care facilities.

J-Curve :A distribution that looks like the letter J or its mirror image when graphed as a frequency polygon.

Jejunum : The part of the small intestine between the duodenum and the ileum, about 8 ft. long.

Jellinek Classification : A classification of alcoholism. *A* psychological, *B* tissue damage but no dependence, *C* fluctuant dependence, *D* constant dependence, *E* bout drinking.

Jelly : A semi-solid substance usually containing gelatin in colloidal solution.

Jet Lag : Physical disorientation of the body when its circadian rhythms are not paralleled by the environmental time of day. It happens when travelling by air through several time zones.

Jet Ventilation : Oxygen mixture blown at high frequency into trachea, producing minimal rise in intrathoracic pressure.

Job Description : A document containing information about a position such as required education or training, experience, lines of authority and designation of experience, as well as a general description of the job and major job objectives.

Jocasta Complex : Sexual attraction of mother towards son. See also *Oedipus Complex*.

Jockey Itch *(Tinea cruris)*. Ringworm of the groin; a fungus infection of the skin of the upper thighs near the genital organs.

JOD : Juvenile-onset diabetes. *Juvenile* relates to childhood or to young persons.

Joint : The point of connection between two or more bones; an articulation.

Joint Mice : Small loose fragments of bone that have become separated within a joint, often the knee.

Joint Probability : The probability of two events both occurring.

Joint Probability Distribution : A probability distribution of two or more random variables.

Judgement Sampling : Non-random (non-probability) sampling.

Judicial Contest : Any controversy that must be decided upon evidence.

Jugular Veins : Any of six veins in the neck, draining blood from the brain, scalp, face and neck.

Jury : A body of individuals legally appointed and sworn to render a verdict on the guilt or innocence of a prisoner or to determine the facts in judicial enquiries.

Juxtaposition : The state of being side by side; the act of placing side by side.

K

Kaiser Criterion : A criterion of determining the number of factors to extract; suggested by Guttman and popularized by Kaiser, also known as the "eigenvalue greater than one" criterion.

Kala-Azar : Visceral leishmaniasis. Irregular fever and emaciation with large liver and spleen, high mortality if untreated.

Kangri Cancer : Skin cancer of lower abdomen in Kashmiris, from use of charcoal braziers beneath clothes.

Kaolin : China clay, hydrated aluminium silicate, used in diarrhoea.

Kaplan-Meier Method : Non-parametric statistical method, used especially for estimating true survival rates without waiting till all subjects have died.

Kappa Statistic : Measure of agreement between two observers, ranging from 0 to 1.

Karman Cannula : A special device used for suction evacuation of uterus in the second month of pregnancy.

Karnofsky Scale : A scale measuring the overall state of a patient, from 10 normal to 1 moribund.

Karyotype : 1.Chromosome constitution of an individual. 2. Picture of chromosomes of one cell sorted into groups.

Kass's Criterion : A measure of urinary infection : 10 pathogens per ml of urine.

Kaye's Test : A test for semen on clothing, measures amount of acid phosphatase in extract.

Kehr's Sign : Shoulder pain in ruptured spleen.

Kell : Blood group system (K, k, etc.) involved in some transfusion reactions and in erythroblastosis.

Kendall's Tau (τ) : A non-parametric measure of correlation that uses ranked data.

Keratitis : Inflammation of the cornea of the eye, causing pain, blurred vision and watery eyes.

Keratoconjunctivitis : Acute inflammation of the cornea and conjunctiva, tending to occur in epidemics, caused by a specific virus.

Keratomalacia : Corneal softening due to vitamin A deficiency.

Keratoplasty : Corneal transplant.

Keratosis : Overgrowth of the horny layer of the skin; for example, a wart or callus.

Kernicterus : A severe form of jaundice characterized by deposits of bile pigments in parts of the brain and degeneration of nerve cells.

Kernig's Sign : Pain on passive straightening of knee with hip flexed, sign of meningitis involving sciatic nerve roots.

Ketosis : Abnormally large amounts of ketone (acetone) bodies in the tissues and fluids; occurs in cases of starvation or Diabetes mellitus.

Keyboard : A set of keys in a typewriter-like arrangement used to enter data or commands into the computer.

Keypunch : A keyboard-operated device that punches holes in a card to represent data.

Kidd : Blood group system (Jk, etc.) involved rarely in transfusion reactions and erythroblastosis.

Kidney Stone : Hard mass of mineral salts (calculus) responsible for *nephrolithiasis*.

Kidney Transplant : Grafting one or two healthy kidneys from a donor into a patient who has kidney failure.

Kinins : Miniature proteins associated with rheumatism and allergic reactions.

Kitemark : Mark or logo which can be displayed by organizations which produce goods, including medical equipment, or deliver services which conform to standards specified by the British Standards Institution; often displayed on products themselves.

Klebsiella : Genus of non-motile coliform bacilli with large capsules and mucoid growth.

Kleptomania : An irresistible desire to steal : mental abnormality associated with depression or stress.

Klinefelter's Syndrome : Undeveloped testes and female characteristics such as breast enlargement in males, due to an abnormality of the sex-determining pair of chromosomes.

Knee Jerk : The patellar reflex; sudden jerking forward of the lower leg when tapped below the kneecap. A test of the integrity of nerves.

Koch's Bacilli : Causative micro-organisms for tuberculosis; a class of bacteria called *Mycobacteria tuberculosis*, or *Koch's bacilli* after Robert Koch, the German bacteriologist.

Koplik's Spots : White spots with red halo, in mouth in early measles.

Krebs Cycle : Citric acid or tricarboxylic acid cycle, mitochondrial system producing energy by acetyl residues.

Kruskal-Wallis Test : A non-parametric test based on ranks that is used to test the hypothesis that three or more independent populations are identical. It is the non-parametric equivalent of the one-way *ANOVA*.

Kurtosis : The degree of the curvature of an unimodal frequency distribution. Kurtosis indicates the extent to which a distribution is more peaked or flat-topped than a normal distribution.

Kwashiorkor : Malnutrition with protein deficiency as the main component, especially as seen after late weaning in African children.

Kyasanur Forest Disease (KFD) : Infection with arbovirus of the togavirus family, tick vector, fever with mild encephalitis, prevalent in South India.

Kyphosis : Excessive backward convexity of spine.

L

Labia : Lips or liplike organs.

Laboratory, Laboratory Technician : Area in the hospital responsible for analyzing samples of blood, urine, tissue, and so on. This lab is staffed by laboratory technicians under the supervision of a pathologist.

Labour : The series of contractions of the uterus prior to the birth of infant.

Laceration : A wound caused by tearing of tissue.

Lacrimal : Pertaining to tears, produced by the *lacrimal gland* in the upper outside region of the eye socket.

Lactation : 1. The secretion of milk. 2. The period of milk secretion.

Lactose : A sugar derived from milk, which on hydrolysis yields glucose and galactose.

Lambda (λ) : The single value needed to define a *Poisson distribution.* It is both the mean and the variance of the distribution.

Laminectomy : Surgery of the wall of the spinal canal to expose underlying structures.

Language : In computer terms, a set of characters, conventions, and rules that is used for conveying information.

Laparoscope : An endoscope for examining the peritoneal cavity.

Laparoscopy : Examination by means of the laparoscope.

Laparotomy : Incision through the flank or, more generally, through any part of the abdominal wall.

Laryngectomy : Surgical removal of all or part of the voice box, usually because of cancer.

Laryngitis : Inflammation of the larynx (the organ of voice).

Laser : A device that amplifies light waves and concentrates them in an intense, penetrating beam; used as a tool in surgery, in diagnosis, and in physiologic studies.

Laser Card : A data recording technique similar to an optical disk but in a card form.

Late Foetal Death : Death of a foetus, after 28 completed weeks' gestation and over 1,001 grams of weight.

Latent : Dormant or concealed; not manifest; potential.

Latent Effect : A confounded effect that results when the effects of previous treatments are re-activated by later treatments.

Latent Funtion : The effect or a result of a pattern of behaviour that is not apparent to the members of society who are engaging in it, *e.g.* funerals to exhibit wealth (*cf. Manifest Function*).

Latent Immunization : The process of developing immunity by a single or repeated inapparent asymptomatic infection.

Latent (Infection) : Persistence of an infectious agent within the host without symptoms (and often without demonstrable presence in blood, tissues, or bodily secretions of the host).

Lateral : Pertaining to a side, away from the midline of the body.

Latin Square : An experimental design that allows two categorical sources of variation to be controlled, while requiring the use of relatively few experimental subjects.

Lavage : The irrigation or washing out of an organ, as of the stomach or bowel.

Laxative : A cathartic or purgative (medicine for purging the bowels).

Lay Reporting : The collection of information, its use, and transmission to other levels of the health system by non-professional, health workers.

L.D.$_{50}$: Median lethal dose. A dose that is lethal for 50% of the test subjects.

Lead Poisoning : Intoxication from absorption of lead or its salts into the body; plumbism.

Lead Time : The time gained in treating or controlling a disease when detection is earlier than usual, *e.g.* in the presymptomatic stage.

Learning Effect : A confounded effect that results when the mere repetition of a treatment or activity changes subjects' responses.

Least Significant Difference : The smallest difference between two group means that would yield a significant result if the two groups were compared using a *t*-test.

Least Squares Criterion : The criterion used in the least squares method to establish a regression line.

Least Squares Method (or Fit) : A method of fitting a calculated trend to statistical data; so called because the sum of the squared deviations of the calculated from the observed variables is a minimum.

Leave of Absence : The authorized absence of an inpatient from a hospital or other inpatient or residential facility for a specified period of time, occurring after admission and prior to discharge.

Legalization : Legal actions that make legal what was previously a criminalized behaviour, product, or condition.

Legitimate Age-specific Birth Rate : Number of legitimate births for a given age group of married women per 1,000 married women in that age group.

Leishmaniasis : A parasitic disease transmitted by sandflies.

Length of Stay : The length of stay for one inpatient or resident is the number of calendar days from admission to discharge.

Leprosy : A chronic communicable disease caused by *Mycobacterium leprae* and characterized by the graunlomatous lesions of the skin, mucous membrane, and peripheral nervous system.

Leptokurtic Distribution : A distribution which is quite peaked or tall—most of the scores occur in the middle of the distribution—with very few scores occurring in the tails.

Leptospirosis : A zoonotic disease caused by a number of the bacterial group known as Leptospira and harboured by many species of lower animals (rats, dogs, cattle, in particular).

Lesbian : A female homosexual.

Lesion : Alteration of tissue or function due to injury or disease.

Leukaemia : Malignant disease of the tissues producing lymphocytes or myelocytes, typically characterized by great increase in the blood of abnormal forms of the respective types of cells.

Leukocytosis : Abnormal increase in numbers of white blood cells.

Leukoderma : An acquired condition with localized loss of pigmentation of the skin.

Leukopenia : Reduction of the number of leukocytes in the blood, the count being 5,000 or less (5×10^9/L).

Leukoplakia : Whitish leathery patches on mucous membranes of the mouth or vulva.

Leukorrhea : A whitish, viscid discharge from the vagina and uterine cavity.

Level of Care : The degree of services and health care available. The degree may be extensive or minimal depending on the health care needs of an individual patient.

Level of Care Criteria : Standards used to determine the appropriate level of care — hospital, skilled nursing facility, intermediate care —for a given patient based on the types of service that can be provided at that level.

Level of Confidence : The extent of certainty about a confidence interval covering the true population mean (proportion).

Level of Significance : A level of probability (usually .05) at which the null hypothesis can be rejected and the research hypothesis can be accepted.

Liability Insurance : Insurance to cover answerable claims, such as malpractice insurance.

Libido : Sexual desire. In psycho-analytical theory, a form of sexual energy with which mental processes, drives, and object-representations are invested.

Licensure : State recognition and authorization to operate.

Licit Drug : A drug that is legally available by medical prescription in the jurisdiction in question, or, sometimes, a drug legally available without medical prescription.

Life Cycle : Term usually employed for multicellular forms of animal life that produce eggs or ova; refers to the usual development sequence from the ovum to the adult capable of producing more ova.

Life Events : Changes or disruptions in the pattern of living that may be associated with, or produce changes in, health (*e.g.* death of a spouse, divorce, loss of job, etc.)

Life Expectancy : Life expectancy, at a given age, is the average number of years which a person at that age is expected to live under the mortality prevalent in the community or country. Life expectancy at birth is used more frequently.

Lifetime Risk : The risk to an individual that a given health effect will occur at any time after exposure, without regard for the time at which that effect occurs.

Life Span : Maximum possible length of life.

Life Style : The set of habits and customs that is influenced, modified, encouraged, or constrained by the lifelong process of socialization.

Life Table : Life history of a group of people, showing such information as the probability of surviving each age period.

Life Table Analysis : A method for analyzing survival times for censored observations that have been grouped into intervals.

Ligament : A band of fibrous tissue connecting bones or cartilages, serving to support and strengthen joints.

Ligature, Ligation : Any material, such as thread or wire, used for tying a vessel or to constrict a part. **Ligation** pertains to the application of ligature.

Likelihood : The probability that a specified sample result will take place, given that a particular state of nature is true.

Likelihood Ratio : In diagnostic testing, the ratio of true-positives to false-positives.

Limbus : A border; the edge of the cornea where it joins the white of the eye.

Limitation of Activity : A long-term reduction in a person's capacity to perform the usual kind or amount of activities associated with his or her age group.

Line Chart : A graph which depicts movement and generally aids the reader in comprehending the trends across time on some variable(s).

Line of Balance : A technique for measuring, collecting, interpreting, and presenting facts—cost, time, and accomplishments — all measured against a specific plan.

Linear Association : The form of a relationship among variables such that when any two variables are plotted, a straight line results.

Linear Combination : A combination in which variables are combined with only constant weights.

Linear Contrast : A weighted combination of group means that reflects some specific question about the nature of the group differences.

Linear Correlation : A measure of the strength of the linear relationship between two variables *y* and *x* that is independent of their respective scales of measurement; commonly measured by the coefficient of correlation.

Linear Programming : A technique of mathematics and operations research for solving certain kinds of problems involving many variables where a best value or set of best values is to be found.

Linear Regression : Procedures for determining the straight line that will help in predicting scores on one variable from scores on another variable, while minimizing the amount of (squared) error.

Linear System : Relationship among variables referred to as a whole, in which all the relationships are linear; factor analysis model in which all of the variables are assumed to be linear functions of underlying factors.

Linkage : In genetics, the association of genes having loci on the same chromosome, which results in the tendency of a group of such genes to be associated in inheritance.

Lipaemia : An excess of lipids (fatty material) in the blood.

Lipids : A broad term for fats and fat-like substances.

Lipoma : A benign fatty tumour usually composed of mature fat cells.

Literacy Rate : The percentage of the population aged 15 and over able to read and write in any language.

Lithiasis : Stones where they don't belong (gallstones, kidney stones); the condition of having stones.

Lithotomy : Cutting into the bladder to remove a stone.

Lithotripsy (Litholapaxy) : The crushing of a stone in the bladder and washing out of the fragments.

Live Birth : A live birth, as defined by the W.H.O. (1993), is "the complete expulsion, irrespective of the duration of the pregnancy, which, after such separation, breaths or shows any other evidence of life, such as beating of the heart, pulsation of the umbilical cord, or definite movement of voluntary muscles, whether or not the umbilical cord has been cut or the placenta is attached".

Live-birth Order : The total number of live-births the mother has had, including the present birth, as recorded on the birth certificate.

Lobectomy : Excision of a lobe, as of the lung, brain, or liver.

Lobotomy : Cutting into a lobe of an organ, especially a lobe of the brain.

Local Area Networks : A high-speed geographically constrained (*e.g.* Hospital 'X') communications arrangement between computing equipment permitting data transfer, sharing of common resources and convenient physical connections to the users.

Location : A computer term signifying a storage position in the main internal storage which can store one computer word and which is usually identified by an address.

Locum (Tenens) : A practitioner who temporarily takes the place of another.

Locus : 1. The position of a point, as defined by coordinates on a graph. 2. The position that a gene occupies on a chromosome.

Lod Score : In genetics, the log odds ratio of observed to expected distribution of genetic markers.

Logarithm (ln) : The exponent indicating the power to which *e* (2.718) is raised to obtain a given number; also called the natural logarithm.

Logic (Symbolic) : The study of formal logic and mathematics by means of a special written language which seeks to avoid the ambiguity and inadequacy of ordinary language.

Logistic Regression : The regression technique used when the outcome is a binary, or dichotomous variable.

Logit : The logarithm of the ratio of frequencies of two different categorical outcomes such as healthy *versus* sick.

Log-linear Analysis : A statistical method for analyzing the relationships among three or more nominal variables.

Logrank Test : A statistical method for comparing two survival curves when there are censored observations.

Longitudinal Health Record : A patient record that includes medical information collected over an extended time, such as a family practice record that includes all medical data on an individual from birth to the present.

Longitudinal Research : A type of post-facto research in which subjects are measured repeatedly throughout their lives in order to obtain data on possible trends in growth and development.

Long-Term Care : Health rendered in a non-acute care facility and to a patient in a resident status; such illness is not severe enough to require an acute care facility but is in need of continued supervision and assistance by health care practitioners.

Loop : A computer term indicating a sequence of instructions that is repeated until a terminal condition prevails.

Lordosis : Forward curvature of the lumbar spine.

Loss Function : A function in terms of the difference between an estimate and the value of the parameter being estimated.

Louse : Any of various parasitic insects (genus : *Pediculus*); major vectors of typhus, relapsing fever, and french fever.

Low Birth Weight (LBW) : A low birth weight is defined as less than 2,500 grams, the measurement being taken within the first hours of life, before significant post-natal weight loss has occurred.

Lower End Limit : The lower end point of a class interval in a grouped frequency distribution.

Lower Tail : The left tail of a distribution.

Lower Tail Probability : A probability calculated by computing an area in the lower tail of a distribution.

LSD : Lysergic acid diethylamide. A chemical compound used in the study of mental disorders and as a psychedelic drug.

Lumbago : Pain in the lumbar (loin) region.

Lumbar Puncture : Withdrawal of cerebrospinal fluid through a hollow needle inserted between lumbar vertebrae of the small of the back.

Lupus : Any of a group of skin diseases in which the lesions are characteristically eroded.

Lymphadenitis : Inflammation of the lymph nodes.

Lymphangitis : Inflammation of lymph vessels due to spread of an infection, producing swelling and burning pain.

Lymphocyte : One of the types of white blood cells; a small round cell which plays a role in immune response, especially in delayed hypersensitivity.

Lymphocytopenia : A reduction of the number of lymphocytes in the blood.

Lysis : Destruction or decomposition, as of a cell or other substances, under influence of a specific agent.

M

Maceration : Softening and deterioration of tissue soaking or in contact with fluids.

Machine : Any combination of mechanisms for utilizing, modifying, applying or transmitting energy, whether simple or complex.

Macrocyte : An abnormally large red blood cell.

Macrocytosis : The state distinguished by the presence of an usually large number of macrocytes in the circulating blood.

Macronutrients : Those food components that supply energy, *i.e.* fats, carbohydrates, proteins and some organic acids.

Macula Lutea : A small, round, yellowish spot near the center of the retina, the area of colour perception and most distinct vision.

Macule : A flat discoloured spot on the surface of the skin.

Mainframe : A computer with a variety of peripheral devices, a large amount of storage, and a fast central processing unit; generally used in comparison with a smaller or subordinate computer.

Maintainability : A characteristic of design and installation which is expressed as the probability that an item can be restored to or retained in satisfactory operating condition within a given period of time when maintenance action is performed in accordance with prescribed procedures and resources.

Major Activity (or Usual Activity) : The principal activity of a person or of his or her age-sex group. For example, for adults 18 years of age and over the major activity usually refers to a job, housework, or school attendance.

Majority : The age which qualifies an individual as legally responsible for his or her own acts; 21 years of age in most countries.

Malaise : A vague and indefinite sensation of not feeling well, of uneasiness or discomfort.

Malaria : A protozoal disease of man, in which the causative organism *Plasmodium,* invades certain body cells and the red blood cells, causing an infection with a characteristic fever pattern.

Malaria Patent Period : Period during which parasites are present in peripheral blood.

Malaria Periodicity : Recurrence at regular intervals of symptoms; periodicity may be quotidian (recurring daily), tertian (recurring every alternate day), or quartan (recurring every fourth day).

Malaria Survey : Investigation in selected age-group samples in randomly selected localities to assess malaria endemicity; uses spleen and/or parasite rates as measures of endemicity.

Malformation : Deformity. Defective or abnormal formation.

Malfunction : Disordered function. To fail to function as it should.

Malignant : Virulent, life threatening.

Malingerer : An individual who deliberately feigns illness or disability for personal gain or to evade obligation.

Malnutrition : Faulty nutrition. Any disorder of nutrition.

Malocclusion : Faulty occlusion or closure of the two rows of teeth.

Malpractice : Failure in the exercise of a reasonable degree of skill and care on the part of a medical practitioner in the treatment of a patient.

Malpresentation : Abnormal presentation of the foetus.

Maltreatment Syndrome : Ongoing pattern of behaviour towards another person, which (a) is outside the norms of conduct, and (b) entails a substantial risk of causing physical or emotional harm.

Mammography : X-ray examination of the breast.

Mammoplasty : Plastic surgery of the breast; especially an operation to correst sagging breasts.

Management : The sum of the measures taken to plan, organize, operate, and evaluate all the many interrelated elements of the system.

Management Data : Data used by management professionals; includes policy and procedure manuals, memos, bylaws, budgets, correspondence, and individual or specialized worksheets developed for individual departmental needs.

Management Service : The application of scientific methods in the study of management, generally through the application of quantitative techniques.

Man-Function : The function allocated to the human component of a system.

Mania : A disorder in which mood is elevated out of keeping with the individual's circumstances and may vary from carefree joviality to almost uncontrollable excitement.

Manic-depressive Insanity : Circular insanity, marked by periodic mania and periodic melancholia.

Manifest Function : The effect or result of a pattern of behaviour that is apparent to the members of a society (*e.g.*, funeral to remove the dead individual, to comfort the mourning family).

Manipulation : The use of forceful passive movements in the treatment of disorders of the joints.

Man/Machine Relationship : Some combination of man and machine working as a well-coordinated team.

Mann-Whitney Test : A non-parametric test of the hypothesis that two independent populations are alike.

Mantel-Haenszel Estimate : An adjusted odds ratio as an estimate of relative risk that may be derived from grouped and matched set of data.

Mantel-Haenszel Test : A summary chi-square test developed by Mantel and Haenszel for stratified data and used when controlling for confounding.

Mantoux Test : One of the tuberculin tests for the diagnosis of tuberculosis, in which the tuberculin is given intracutaneously.

Marasmus : Progressive wasting, especially in infants, for which there is no specific cause.

Marginal Frequencies (Probabilities) : The row and column frequencies (or probabilities) in a contingency table; *i.e.* the frequencies listed on the margins of the table.

Marginal Utility : Satisfaction derived from the last or additional expenditure. Additional increments of expenditure for a given product tend to result in declining additions of utility.

Marijuana (Marihuana) : See *Cannabis*.

Marital Status : The status of an individual whether married or unmarried. The former includes all married people, including those separated from their spouces, and the latter includes those who are single (never married), divorced, or widowed.

Marrow : The soft pulpy tissue in the hollows of the long bones and in the spaces of the spongy substance of all tissues.

Masculinization : The induction or development of male secondary sex characteristics in the female.

Masochism : A form of sexual perversion in which sexual excitement and pleasure are enhanced by being simultaneously beaten or humiliated.

Massage : The method of physiotherapy characterized by a varying combination of rubbing, kneading, tapping, pinching and manipulation.

Mastectomy : Excision or amputation of the breast.

Master Patient Index : A condensed list of data that provides identification and location information regarding medical or health records.

Mastitis : Inflammation of the breasts, from bacterial infection or other causes.

Mastodynia : Pain in the breast.

Masturbation : Production of an orgasm by self-manipulation of the genitals.

Match Rate : The proportion of records from a given data collection system that are found to match the records of another system.

Matched Samples : Samples such that each element in one sample is paired with one element in the other sample.

Matched *t*-Test : Procedures for testing hypotheses about the difference between two population means, using matched samples.

Matching Rules : A set of criteria used to determine whether or not two records are a match—that is, whether they are to be treated as referring to the same person or event.

Matching Status : The classification of a record in relation to the final outcome of a matching process—that is, whether a particular record is a match or a non-match.

Materia Medica : The branch of medical science that deals with the sources, preparation and uses of drugs.

Maternal Death : The death of a woman while pregnant or within 42 days of termination of pregnancy, irrespective of the duration and the site of the pregnancy, from any cause related to or aggravated by the pregnancy or its management, but not from accidental or incidental causes.

Maternal Mortality Rate : The number of maternal deaths attributed to complications of pregnancy and childbirth occurring over a year, divided by the total number of live-births in the year; often expressed as the number of maternal deaths per 1,000 live-births.

Maternity Floor/Ward/Wing : The part of the hospital where mothers give birth to babies and are cared for afterward.

Mathematical Models : Mathematical formulations that attempt to describe, predict or to control real-world phenomena.

Mauchly's Test : A test used in repeated-measures analysis of variance to determine whether the variance-co-variance assumptions of the univariate approach hold.

Maximum Criterion : A decision procedure that chooses an act that yields the maximum of the minimum pay-offs.

Maximum Likelihood Solution : A method of statistical estimation which seeks to identify the population parameters with a maximum likelihood of generating the observed sample distribution.

McNemar Test : Technique developed by the statistician Quinn McNemar that uses chi-square for the analysis of nominal data from correlated samples.

Mean : The most common measure of central tendency, equal to the sum of the observed qualities divided by the number of observed quantities.

Mean Duration of Life : Expectation of life at birth.

Mean Effects : When two or more independent variables are involved (as in an ANOVA), the mean effects are produced by the action of each independent variable working separately.

Mean Square (MS) : In ANOVA, a sum of squares divided by its degrees of freedom.

Mean Square Error : A measure of total error, equal to the sum of the variance and the square of the bias.

Measles : An acute infectious disease, caused by a virus, and with a characteristic rash.

Measure of Association : A number whose magnitude indicates the degree of correspondence — *i.e.* strength of relationship—between two variables.

Measures of Central Tendency : Index or summary numbers that describe the middle of a distribution. See *Mean, Medium, Mode.*

Measures of Dispersion : Index or summary numbers that describe the spread of observations about the mean. See *Range, Standard Deviation.*

Measure of Effectiveness : The quantitative expression used to compare the utility of an alternative in achieving an objective.

Measurement : A method of quantifying observations by assigning numbers to them on the basis of specific rules, thus facilitating comparison with standards.

Measurement Scale : The complete range of possible values for a measurement; classified into five major types : dichotomous, nominal, ordinal, interval, and ratio.

Measurement Validity : The absence of random and/or systematic measurement error.

Meatotomy : Surgical incision of the urinary meatus in order to enlarge it.

Meconium : The first faecal discharge of the new-born infant, consisting of bile, intestinal debris, and mucus.

Median : Middle. The mid-point that divides the area of a frequency curve into two halves.

Median Length of Life : Age by which half of the original members of a cohort have died (synonym : *Probable Lifetime*).

Medicaid : The U.S. federal health programme designed for the recipients of categorical aid programmes. *i.e.* the medically indigent (poor, needy).

Medical Administration : The management of affairs relevant to the practice of medicine.

Medical Advisory Board : A standing or permanent committee (comprising the medical director, the hospital administrator, and selected physicians) that advises the hospital board on general medical policies; and reviews the performance of physicians; also referred to as the *Joint Conference Committee.*

Medical Audit : Professional evaluation of the quality of medical care offered to patients.

Medical Audit Committee : Committee responsible for evaluation of the quality of care provided to patients by the medical and other professional staff who are directly responsible for patient care.

Medical Care Evaluation : A structured programme to measure the quality of care given to patients; encompasses such measurement functions as audit, appraisal, peer review, quality assurance, etc.

Medical Care Outcome : The end result of a patient's state of illness during an episode of treatment or a period of care during chronic illness.

Medical Care Unit : An assemblage of patient beds and related facilities and assigned personnel in which medical services are provided to a defined and limited class of patients according to their particular medical care needs.

Medical Classification System : A method of arranging like or related disease entities in groups for the reporting of quantitative data for statistical purposes.

Medical Consultation : See *Consultation.*

Medical Decision Making (or Analysis) : The application of probabilities to the decision process in medicine; the basis for cost-benefit analysis.

Medical Department : A division of medical services in the hospital that offers diagnosis and treatment in one area (*e.g.* surgery, neurology, paediatrics).

Medical Director : The physician responsible for the medical services in the hospital; usually appointed by the hospital board and advised by members of the medical staff; sometimes referred to as the *Chief of Staff.*

Medical Effectiveness (Validity) : The clinically proved efficacy of a specific treatment, test, etc. in terms of patient outcome.

Medical Record : A permanent document on which everything relating to a patient's medical diagnosis and treatment during his/her hospital stay is recorded.

Medical Record Administrator : The individual responsible for developing and directing the objectives and activities that comprise an information system to compile and distribute patient data.

Medical Record Committee : Committee which sees that accurate and complete medical records are developed and retained for every patient treated.

Medical Social Workers : Professionals working in co-operation with the medical staff to assist patients with personal problems such as home or work conditions, provision for dependents etc., which may create difficulties during illness.

Medical Staff : Qualified medical personnel responsible for the quality of all medical care provided to patients and for the ethical conduct and professional practices of individual physicians.

Medical Staff Bylaws : Rules and regulations which define duties, qualifications, and method of selection of officers of the medical staff.

Medical Terminology : The study of words used to communicate facts and ideas particular to medicine.

Medicament : A medicinal agent.

Medicare : A programme of the U.S. Social Security Administration which provides medical care to the aged.

Medication : 1. A medicament. 2. The administration of remedies. 3. Impregnation with a medicine.

Medicine : 1. A drug. 2. The healing art. 3. The non-surgical practice of the healing art.

Medicolegal : Pertaining to medicine and the law.

MEDLARS : *Medical Literature Analysis and Retrieval System* : a computer-based system derived from journals indexed for *Index Medicus, Index to Dental Literature,* and the *International Nursing Index.*

MEDLINE : MEDLARS on-line; a shortened form of the MEDLARS system.

Megabyte : 1024 × 1024 or 1,048,576 bytes, approximately one million bytes.

Megalomania : The condition characterized by delusions of grandeur.

Melena : The passage of dark, tarry stools, containing altered blood due to bleeding in the stomach or upper part of the intestines.

Melancholia : A mental illness characterized by extreme depression or black despair.

Melanin : A yellowish to black pigment which is a factor in skin colour.

Melanoma : A tumour composed of pigmented cells.

Memory Cycle : A computer term for 1. The process of reading and restoring information in magnetic core memory. 2. The time required to complete this process.

Menarche : The establishment of menstruation.

Meningitis : Inflammation of the meninges (the membranes that surround the brain and spinal cord).

Menopause : The cessation of menstruation at the end of reproductive life.

Menorrhagia : Excessive loss of blood during menstruation.

Menses : The monthly flow of blood at menstruation.

Menstruation : The periodic uterine bleeding which occurs throughout the sexually active period of a woman's life.

Mental Disorder : An imprecise term designating any disorder of the mind, acquired or congenital.

Mental Health Organization : An institution or agency whose primary concern is the provision of direct mental health services to the mentally ill or emotionally disturbed.

Mental Retardation : A condition of arrested or incomplete development of the mind, characterized by impairment of skills manifested during the developmental period, contributing to the overall level of intelligence.

Menu Driven : A programme whose use is controlled by a series of menus.

Mesokurtic : A unimodal frequency distribution whose curve is normal.

Mesomorph : A person of medium height and stocky build.

Meta-Analysis : A method for combining the results from several independent studies of the same outcome so that an overall *P*-value may be determined.

Metabolism : The chemical and physical changes, whereby the living lives, moves and has its being.

Metastasis : The transfer of disease from one part of the body to another not directly connected with it, as occurs, for example, in the case of cancer.

Metatarsalgia : Foot pain in the instep area, usually due to weakness of muscles and ill-fitting shoes.

Methadone : A synthetic opiate drug used in maintenance therapy for those dependent on opioids. It has a long half-life, and can be given orally once daily with supervision.

Methanol, Methyl Alcohol : A widely used industrial solvent. When ingested it is highly toxic, causing blindness. Also known as wood alcohol.

Method of Study, Methodology : The general pattern (or blueprint) for organizing the procedures for gathering and analyzing all the data for an investigation.

Method Study : A study with the specific aim of developing new data collection methods or analytical techniques.

Metritis : Inflammation of the uterus.

Metrorrhagia : Abnormal bleeding from the uterus at times other than the menstrual period.

Microbe : A unique, unicellular living organism, especially a pathogenic bacterium.

Microbiology : A science dealing with the study of micro-organisms.

Microcephaly : Congenital smallness of the head, with defective development of the brain and premature ossification of the skull.

Microcomputer : A complete small computer system built around a microprocessor CPU.

Microfiche : A microscopic photographic copy of text or graphic data.

Microfilming : A process of photographing and reducing a given report to a miniature of the original on film.

Microgram : One-thousandth part of a milligram (Abbreviation : μ g; mcg. in prescriptions).

Micronutrients : Chemical agents and organic molecules that cannot be synthesized through human metabolism but which are essential for metabolic function (*e.g.* zinc, iodine, folic acid).

Microscope : An instrument for magnifying objects and revealing details of structure not otherwise distinguishable.

Microtome : An instrument for cutting sections for microscopy.

Micturition : The act of voiding urine. Urination.

Mid-point : The value halfway between the lower real limit and the upper limit of a class interval.

Midwife : A person who is qualified to supervise women in childbirth.

Migraine : A condition characterized by recurring unilateral, frontal or temporal headaches, accompanied by visual disturbances and nausea and/or vomiting.

Migrant : In demography, a person whose change of residence takes him into a different politico-geographic unit.

Migrant Studies : Studies taking advantage of migration to one country by those from other countries with different physical and biological environments, cultural background and/or genetic makeup, and different morbidity or mortality experience.

Migration : Movement of people from one geographical location to another within the same country or across country borders.

Milestone, Delayed : Failure to achieve an expected level of development by the age at which it is ordinarily achieved.

Miliaria : Prickly heat, heat rash.

Minicomputer : A computer whose size, speed and capability lie in between a mainframe and a microcomputer.

Miscarriage : Abortion. Premature expulsion of the fertilized ovum before the foetus is viable; *i.e.* before the 28th week of pregnancy.

Mismatch : The linkage of a record from one system that has a partner in the other system with the wrong record in the second system.

Missing Data : Information that is not available for a particular case (*e.g.* a person) for which at least some other information is available.

Misuse (Drug, Alcohol) : Use of a substance for a purpose not consistent with legal or medical guidelines, as in the non-medical use of prescription medicines.

Mittelschmerz : Pain midway between the menstrual periods.

Mobility, Geographic : Movement of persons from one country or region to another.

Mobility, Patient : Ability of a patient to go outdoors, assessed with mechanical aid if customarily used.

Mobility, Social : Movement from one defined socio-economic group to another, either upward or downward.

Modal Class : The class in a frequency distribution that occurs more in observations than any other.

Modal Number : The most frequent number in a distribution.

Mode : The value that occurs with the greatest frequency.

Model: A simplified representation of an operation containing only those aspects of primary importance to the problem under study.

Modem : *Mo*dulator-*Dem*odulator. A device at each end of an analog communications line for translating digital signals into analog form and *vice versa*.

Modernization : The process of social change whereby less developed societies acquire characteristics common to more developed societies, accompanied by rapid economic growth.

Module : A small programme which can be compiled separately and linked to form part of a large programme.

Mole : 1. A localized aggregation of naevus cells. 2. A degenerative mass in the uterus. 3. A chemical unit.

Mongolism : Down's syndrome. The congenital form of mental subnormality, due to chromosomal abnormality, and associated with characteristic physical defects.

Moniliasis : Infection caused by yeast like organisms, usually *Candida albicans,* which have a predilection for mucous membranes.

Monitor : A functional unit that observes and records selected activities within a data processing system for analysis.

Monitoring : The continuous follow-up of activities to ensure that they are proceeding according to plan.

Monte Carlo Method : Any procedure that involves statistical sampling techniques from a distribution of possible outcomes for obtaining a probabilistic approximation to the solution of a physical or mathematical problem.

Morbidity : The incidence and/or prevalence of certain diseases or disabilities in the community.

Morbidity Rate : The number of cases of disease per 1,000 persons at risk (term used indiscriminately to refer to incidence or prevalence rates of diseases.)

Morbidity Survey : A method for estimating the prevalence and/or incidence of disease or diseases in a population.

Moribund : In the state of dying.

Moron : A feeble-minded person whose "mental age" is between 8 and 12 years.

Morphine : A powerful narcotic analgesic, characterized by the rapid development of dependence and habituation; the principal alkaloid of opium.

Morphology : The science of organic forms and structure.

Mortality : Deaths or death rates, in a community.

Mortality Rate : The number of deaths in a defined population over a specified period of time. It is the number of people who die during a given period of time divided by the number of people at risk during the period.

Mortality Statistics : Statistical tables compiled from the information contained in death certificates; usually show numbers of deaths and/or rates by age, sex, cause, and sometimes other variables.

Mortuary : A building in which the dead are placed awaiting burial or disposal.

Motion Sickness : Nausea and vomiting induced by forms of motion (sea sickness, car sickness, air sickness).

MOU : *M*emorandum *O*f *U*nderstanding. A signed statement outlining, the responsibilities of each party involved.

Mountain Sickness : A temporary condition brought on by diminished amounts of oxygen in the air at high altitudes.

Mouse : An input device with which the cursor can be moved on the screen by moving the mouse over a flat surface.

Mover : In demography a person who changes his place of residence.

Moving Average : A series of averages used to reduce irregularities in a time series by selecting a set number of successive items in the series, computing the average, then dropping the first item and adding the next succeeding one, etc.; used to average out random movements and, thereby, reveal underlying trends.

MS-DOS : *M*icrosoft-*D*isc *O*perating *S*ystem. An operating system for microcomputers developed by *Microsoft* and in a slightly different version for the IBM-PC.

Mucolytic : Possessing the property of destroying mucus.

Mull : The process of thinking about the data and techniques of a study.

Multicollinearity : A condition in which two or more of the independent variables are strongly (but not perfectly) related to one another in a linear relationship.

Multigravida : A woman who is bearing her second or subsequent child.

Multimodal Distribution : Data distribution with more than one mode. Distribution with two modes are *bimodal.*

Multinomial Distribution : The generalization of the binomial distribution for the situation of more than two possible outcomes on each trial.

Multipara : A woman who has borne two or more children.

Multiple Birth : Two or more babies delivered without complications.

Multiple Comparisons : Comparisons resulting from many statistical tests performed for the same observations.

Multiple Causation : The concept that a given disease may have more than one cause. A combination of causes may be required to produce the effect.

Multiple R : A single numerical value that quantifies the correlations among three or more variables.

Multiple Regression : Technique using the multiple R for making predictions of one variable given measures on two or more others.

Multiplicity Problem : The tendency for a large number of tests to lead to rejection of some of the null hypotheses even when all of the null hypotheses are true.

Multisectoral Action : Action in which the health sector and other relevant sectors collaborate for the achievement of a common goal, the contributions of the different sectors being closely coordinated (synonym : *Intersectoral Action*).

Multivariate Analysis : Any analytic method that allows the simultaneous study of two or more dependent variables.

Multivariate Analysis of Variance (MANOVA) : An advanced statistical method that provides a global test when there are multiple dependent variables and the independent variables are nominal; analogous to ANOVA with multiple outcome measures.

Multivariate Normality : A type of distribution for a group of random variables that implies that each random variable has a normal distribution.

Mummification : Drying and shrivelling of tissue to a mummy-like mass, a result of dry gangrene.

Mumps : A virus infection involving primarily the parotid glands. Epidemic parotitis.

Munchausen Syndrome : Habitual seeking of hospital treatment for apparent acute illness, the patient giving a plausible and dramatic history, all of which is false.

Murmur : A sound of varying intensity, pitch and character based on auscultation over the heart.

Mutation : Change in genetically determined character.

Mutation Rate : The frequency with which mutations occur per gene or per generation.

Mutually Exclusive Events : Two or more events for which the occurrence of one event precludes the occurrence of the others.

Myasthenia Gravis : A chronic debilitating disease characterized by rapid fatigue of certain muscles, with prolonged time of recovery of function.

Mycoses : Infections caused by fungi.

Myelitis : Inflammation of the spinal cord or bone marrow.

Myelogram : An X-ray film of the spinal canal made after injecting a contrast medium opaque to X-rays.

Myocarditis : Inflammatory disease of the heart muscle.

Myringitis: Inflammation of the tympanic membrane (or myringa).

Myringoplasty : Plastic repair of a perforation in the tympanic membrane.

Myxoedema : Adult hypothyroidism, characterized by mental and physical lethargy, dry skin, puffy face, and a low basal metabolic rate.

N

Naevus : A developmental blemish of the skin (usually circumscribed) which is not due to external causes.

Narcolepsy : A paroxysmal disorder with a hereditary basis characterized by a sudden irresistible tendency to fall asleep, usually for brief periods.

Narcosis : A state of deep sleep, unconsciousness, and insensitivitiy to pain.

Narcotic : A chemical agent that induces stupor, coma, or insensibility to pain.

National Health Council : A national body set up to advise a government on health and related socio-economic issues for the entire country.

National Health Expenditure : A measure that estimates the amount spent for all health services and supplies and health-related research and construction activities consumed in a nation during the calendar year.

National Health Policy : A set of decisions to pursue courses of action aimed at achieving defined goals for improving the health situation of a nation.

National Health Strategy : Broad lines of action required in all the sectors concerned to give effect to the national health policy, indicating the problems and ways of dealing with them.

National Plan of Action (Health) : A broad intersectoral master plan for implementing the strategy in order to attain the national health goals.

Natural Growth : Change in population as a result of births and deaths, and excluding migration.

Natural History (of a disease) : Comprehensive account of the nature of the agent, its sources and distribution, mechanisms and its impact on man. In other words, the epidemiology of a disease.

Naturopathy : A form of therapy that avoids medicinal and surgical agencies, and utilizes the so-called natural forces such as heat and massage.

Nausea : The sensation of sickness without actual vomiting.

Necrophilia : Morbid attraction to death or to dead bodies; sexual intercourse with a dead body.

Necropsy : A post-mortem examination.

Necrosis : Circumscribed death of cells or tissue with structural evidence of death.

Negative Correlation : Linear association of increasing values of one variable with decreasing values of another variable.

Negatively Skewed Distribution : A distribution with some extremely low scores, resulting in a frequency polygon with a pronounced tail at the left.

Negligence : Failure to exercise the reasonable prudent care that the circumstances justly demand.

Negotiation : A form of interaction through which individuals, organizations, and governments try to arrange a new combination of some of their common and conflicting interests.

Nematode : A roundworm; any individual of the class Nematoda (a class of helminths, many of which are parasites).

Neonatal Death : The death of a liveborn infant within the first 28 days from the moment of birth.

Neonatal Mortality Rates : The number of children who die in the neonatal period (up to 28 days after birth) during a stated year per 1,000 live births occurring in the same year.

Neonatal Period : The part of an infant's life from the hour of birth through the first 28 days of life. During this period the infant is referred to as a newborn infant.

Neonate : A new-born infant.

Neoplasm : A tumour. Any new or abnormal growth in which cell multiplication is uncontrolled and progressive; may be benign or malignant.

Nephrectomy : Surgical removal of a kidney.

Nephritis : Inflammation of the kidney.

Nephrolithotomy : The surgical removal of a renal stone by means of incising the kidney.

Nephrology : The branch of medical science that deals with the kidneys.

Nephroma : Malignant tumour of the cortex of the kidney.

Nephropexy : Surgical anchoring of a "loose" or floating kidney.

Nephrosis : A degenerative condition of the kidney, characterized by gross albuminuria, oedema and anaemia.

Nephrotoxic : Poisonous to the kidneys.

Nerve Deafness : Impairment of hearing from failure of auditory nerves to transmit impulses to hearing centers in the brain.

Net Autopsy Rate : The ratio during any given period of time of all inpatient autopsies to all inpatient deaths minus coroners' or medical examiners' cases.

Net Migration : The difference (positive or negative) between in- and out-migration (*i.e.* immigration and emigration); also known as *Balance of Migration.*

Net Migration Rate : The net effect of immigration and emigration on an area's population expressed as an increase or decrease per 1,000 population of the area in a given year.

Net Nuptiality : Double decrement table taking account of attrition both through change of marital status and through death.

Net Regression Coefficient : Slope coefficient *(b* value) in multiple regression analysis.

Net Reproduction Rate (NRR) : A measure of the number of live daughters that would be born to a group of newborn girls if up to the end of their reproductive age span they were exposed to the same mortality rates by age and bore daughters at the same rate by age as all women in a given year.

Network : A set of computers and peripherals connected by communications links.

Neuralgia : Pain in the course or distribution of a nerve.

Neuraesthenia : Nervous exhaustion. A neurosis characterized by mental and physical irritability and a sense of fatigue.

Neuritis : Inflammation of a nerve or its parts due to infection, toxins, compression or other causes.

Neurogenic : Of nervous origin.

Neuroleptic : One of a class of drugs used for the treatment of acute and chronic psychoses. Also known as major tranquillizers and antipsychotics.

Neurology : The branch of medicine dealing with the nervous system and its disorders.

Neuromuscular : Pertaining to nerves and muscles.

Neuropathy, Peripheral : Disorder and functional disturbance of the peripheral nerves, manifested as numbness of the extremities, paraesthenia, weakness of the limbs, and loss of deep tendon reflexes.

Neurosis : A mental or emotional disturbance, usually manifesting itself by some functional disturbance of the body without any structural lesion.

Neurosurgery : Surgery of the nervous system.

Neurotic : Relating to a neurosis or an individual suffering from a neurosis. An unduly highly strong person.

Neurotoxic : Having a toxic effect on nervous tissue.

Newman-Keuls Procedure : A multiple comparison method for making pairwise comparisons between means following a significant *F* test in analysis of variance.

Nicotine : The major psychoactive alkaloid substance in tobacco, having both stimulant and relaxing effects.

Nidation : "Nesting"; implantation of a fertilized egg in the uterus.

Nidus : 1. A focus of infection. 2. The site of origin of a pathological process.

Night Blindness (nyctalopia) : Imperfect vision at the night or in dim light; reduced dark adaptation.

Night Nurse : Nurse who works on the night shift.

Ninty-five Per cent Confidence Interval : The range of mean values (proportions) within which there are 95 chances out of 100 that the true population mean (proportion) will fall.

Nitrous Oxide : Laughing gas. A short-acting general anaesthetic, used widely in dentistry and obstetrics.

Nocturia : Excessive urination at night.

Node : In computer terminology, a station on a network where one or more devices can be connected.

Noise : An electronics term referring to disturbing electrical impulses within the audio range, introduced in a circuit by equipment components, man's interference or natural disturbance.

Nomenclature, Medical : A recognized system of preferred terminology for naming disease processes.

Nominal (or Categorical) Data : Data (measurements) in which numbers are used to label discrete, mutually exclusive categories.

Nominal (or Categorical) Scale : The simplest scale of measurement; used for characteristics that have no numerical values (for example, race and gender); also called a *Qualitative Scale*.

Nomogram : A form of line chart showing scales for the variables included in a particular formula in such a way that corresponding values for each variable lie on a straight line intersecting all the scales.

Non-compos Mentis : Of unsound mind, including all forms of mental unsoundness.

Non-mutually Exclusive Events : Two or more events for which the occurrence of one event does not preclude the occurrence of the others.

Non-linear Relationship : When the form of the model describing y in terms of x is not a straight line.

Non-parametric Tests : A family of statistical tests (also called distribution-free tests) that do not require any assumptions about the distribution the data set follows and that do not require the testing of distribution parameters such as means or variance.

Non-participants (or Non-responders) : Members of a study sample or population who do not take part in the study for whatever reasons, or members of a target population who do not participate in an activity.

Non-patient Revenue : Revenues received for which no direct patient care services are rendered. The most widely recognized source of non-patient revenues is philanthropy.

Non-physician Health Care Providers : Those health professionals who do not hold a doctor of medicine degree but are qualified by education or licensure to practice a profession and are involved in direct patient care services.

Non-probability Sample : A sample selected in such a way that the probability that a subject is selected, is unknown.

Non-randomized Trial : A clinical trial in which subjects are assigned to treatments on other than a randomized basis. It is subject to several biases.

Non-response : In a sample survey the failure to obtain information from a designated element for any reason.

Non-standard Normal Distribution : A normal distribution with a mean other that 0 or a standard deviation other than 1.

Non-viable : Incapable of living.

Normal Delivery : A baby delivered without complications.

Normal Distribution : A symmetric, bell-shaped probability distribution with mean μ and standard deviation σ. If observations follow a normal distribution, the interval $(\mu - 2\sigma)$ contains 95% of the observations. Also called the *Gaussian Distribution.*

Normal-Form Analysis : Preposterior analysis carried out by a comparison of the net payoffs of all possible strategies.

Normal Values : Values regarded as being within the usual range of variation in a given population or population sub-group. The range of such values is called the *normal range.*

Normative : Pertaining to the normal, usual, accepted standard or values.

Normative Criteria : Opinions of experts, as to what constitutes good care.

Norms : Numerical or statistical measures of usually observed performance.

Nosocomial Infection : An infection occurring in a patient in a hospital or other health care facility and in whom it was not present at the time of admission; includes infections acquired in the hospital but appearing after discharge, and also such infections among the staff and visitors of the facility.

Nosology : The science of the classification of diseases.

Notation, Binary : A number system written to the base two notation.

Notifiable Disease : A disease that by statutory requirements, must be reported to the public health authority in the pertinent jurisdiction when the diagnosis is made.

Notional Sampling Frame : A sampling frame in which the target population can be defined but the individuals that constitute this population cannot (for example, all individuals who will use a particular hospital emergency room in the next month.)

Nuchal : Pertaining to or in the region of the nape of the neck.

Nuclear Family : A family consisting of the head of the household, spouse and unmarried children living together.

Nuclear Medicine : The application of radioactive materials to diagnosis and treatment and the study of human disease.

Nullipara : A woman who has not borne children.

Null Hypothesis : The initial assumption that the results are simply due to chance, *i.e.* no effect is actually present in the study (for example, that two drugs being compared are equally effective).

Number Index : A chronological listing of all numbers issued with cross references to the names of the patients to which the numbers have been assigned.

Numbering System : An identifying method that utilizes assigned numbers to label each record for filing in a systematic manner for easy retention and retrieval.

Numerator : That number representing the actual number of conditions, individuals, and events counted; the part of the fraction above the line.

Numerical Scale : The highest level of measurement; used for characteristics that can be given numerical values; the differences between numbers have meaning (examples are height, weight, blood pressure); also called *Interval* or *Ratio Scale.*

Nurse : 1. One who looks after the sick or an infant. 2. To take care of the sick. 3. To suckle.

Nurse-midwife : A fully accredited nurse trained to handle uncomplicated delivery of babies and to examine women and prescribe birth control methods.

Nursery : The place in which newborn babies are cared for after their delivery. **Premature Nursery** : A nursery for babies who are born before the end of the normal nine-month gestation period.

Nurse's Aid : A person without a formal nursing degree who assists the nursing staff.

Nurse's Station : A central area on the floor or ward where nurses are based.

Nursing Care : Provision of any of the following services : application of dressings or bandages; bowel and bladder retraining; catheterization; enema; full bed bath; hypodermic, intramuscular, or intravenous injection; irrigation; nasal feeding; oxygen therapy; and temperature-pulse-respiration or blood pressure measurement.

Nursing Home : An establishment with three or more beds that provides nursing or personal care services to the aged, infirm, or clinically ill.

Nutrition : The sum of the processes involved in the ingestion and absorption of food.

Nyctalopia : See *Night Blindness*.

Nymphomania : Insatiable sexual desire of a female.

Nystagamus : Involuntary, rhythmic oscillation of the eyeballs, horizontal, vertical, or rotary.

O

Obesity : Fatness. An excessive accumulation of weight.

Objective : Not influenced by the personal prejudices or feelings of the subject or researcher; unbiased.

Objective Function : A mathematical statement of goals, usually profit maximization.

Objective Probability : An estimate of probability from observable events or phenomena.

Objectives : The end results a programme seeks to achieve (for example, the objectives of health education will be to ensure that people will want to be healthy, know how to stay healthy, do what they can individually and collectively to maintain health, and know how to seek help when required).

Oblimax : A criterion for obtaining an oblique rotation : it is equivalent to the quartimax criterion in orthogonal rotation.

Oblimin : A general criterion for obtaining an oblique rotation which tries to simplify the pattern matrix by way of reference axes.

Oblique Factors : Factors that are correlated with each other; factors obtained through oblique rotation.

Oblique Rotation : The operation through which a simple structure is sought; factors are rotated without imposing the orthogonality condition and resulting terminal factors are correlated with each other.

Observational Studies : Studies (often called surveys) in which the behaviour of the subjects is merely observed and no attempt is made to impose intervention on them.

Observation (Information) Bias : An attribute of data collection. In the collection of data from two groups (cases, controls; exposed, non-exposed) observation bias occurs when non-comparable methods of data collection are used.

Observation Patient : A patient who presents with a medical condition with a significant degree of inability and patient disability, who needs to be monitored, evaluated and assessed for admission to inpatient status or discharged for care in another setting.

Observed Values : The number of individuals actually observed in practice in the various categories of a categorical variable.

Obsession : A fixed idea that cannot be eliminated by reasoning.

Obstetrician : One who practices obstetrics.

Obstetrics : The branch of medicine dealing with pregnancy, labour, and the puerperium.

Obtained Frequencies : In a chi-square analysis the results that are actually obtained when conducting a study.

Occasion of Service : A specific identifiable act of service provided a patient, such as performance of a test, medical examination, treatment or procedure.

Occlusion : The act of closing or being closed.

Occult : Hidden, not evident to the naked eye; as occult blood in faeces.

Occupancy Per cent, Occupancy Ratio : See *Bed Occupancy Ratio.*

Occupational Therapy : A method for the treatment of physical or psychological impairments, based on purposeful occupation and aiming to restore motivation, confidence, and specific skills.

Occurrence Screening : System for selecting cases from hospital records for subsequent review. (Screening personnel have lists of criteria —often adverse occurrences—for selection.)

Ocular : Pertaining to the eye.

Oculist : Same as ophthalmogist.

Odds Ratio : The ratio of the probability that an event will occur to the probability that the event will not occur (for example, the odds of having the disease among the exposed divided by the odds of having the disease among the non-exposed).

Oedema : Dropsical swelling due to an excess of fluid in the intercellular tissues.

Oedipus Complex : Abnormal attachment of a child to the parent of the opposite sex, with an accompanying hostility to the parent of the same sex.

Office Automation : The use of computer based technology to increase the productiviry of office workers.

Office Visit : Any direct personal exchange between an ambulatory patient and a physician or members of his or her staff for the purpose of seeking care and rendering health services.

Off-line : A computer term pertaining to the operation of a functional unit when not under the direct control of the computer.

Off-line Quality Control : Statistical techniques, especially experimental design methods, used in quality control to improve the design of a product.

Ogive : The graph of a cumulative frequency distribution.

Ointment : A semisolid preparation consisting of a fatty substance mixed with an active drug, for external use.

Olfactory : Associated, or to do, with the sense of smell.

Oligomenorrhea : Scanty menstrual flow, or abnormally long time between menstrual periods.

Oligospermia : Abnormally low number of spermatozoa in the semen.

Oliguria : Abnormally low excretion of urine.

Omega-Squared (ω^2) : A statistic that estimates the effect size in the population.

Omphalic : Pertaining to the navel.

Omphalotomy : Cutting of the umbilical cord.

Omentum : A fold of pritoneum, extending between abdominal organs.

On Call : Available for duty but not actually at work. A health care professional who is on call is usually at home, but he/she will come to the hospital if needed.

Oncology : The study of new growths or tumours.

On Duty : Term used to refer to the time when an employee is at work. The opposite is *off duty*.

One-day Surgery : See *Ambulatory Surgery*.

One Per cent Level of Significance (P<0.01) : A level of probability at which the null hypothesis is rejected if an obtained sample difference occurs by chance only 1 time or less out of 100.

One-sample *t*-Test : A statistical test of the hypothesis that the population mean is equal to some hypothesized value.

One-sample Tests : Tests of hypotheses based on data contained in a single sample.

One-Sided Alternative : A test in which the null hypothesis is rejected by observing a statistic that falls in one tail of the appropriate sampling distribution.

One-tailed Test : A test in which the alternative hypothesis specifies a deviation from the null hypothesis in one direction only. The critical region is located in one end of the distribution of the test statistic; also called a *Directional Test.*

One-way ANOVA : A statistical test (*F* test) used to compute several sample means to determine if one or more have come from populations with different means. Used only with research designs with one independent variable.

On-line Patient Records : Computerized patient records stored on a storage device which permits direct, immediate access through terminals.

On-line Processing : Processing performed on equipment directly under the control of the central processor, while the user remains in communication with the computer.

On-line Quality Control : The use of statistical methods, especially control charts, to monitor the consistency of manufactured products.

Onychia : Inflammation of the bed of a nail, often resulting in loss of the nail.

Onychophagy : Nail-biting.

Oophorectomy : Surgical excision of an ovary.

Open Birth Interval : Interval between last birth and the date of the study.

Open-ended Group : An age group, or other classification, that has no definite limit at one end (for example, age 65+).

Open-ended Questions : Questions that must be answered with a sentence, or several sentences.

Operating Characteristic Curve : A plot of the probability of accepting the null hypothesis when some alternative is true (the probability of a Type II error) against various possible values of the alternative hypothesis.

Operating Physician : The clinician who performs the Principal Procedure (which see).

Operating Room (Theatre) : An area of a hospital equipped and staffed to provide facilities and personnel services for the performance of surgical procedures.

Operating System : In computer terminology, software for controlling the execution of computer programmes that may provide scheduling, debugging, input/output control, accounting, compilation, storage allocation, data management, and related services.

Operation : Any action performed with instruments or by the hands of a surgeon; a surgical procedure.

Operational Definition : A description or actual display of a process, action, or object suggested as an analogue or single representative example of what is meant by the term being defined.

Operations Research : The use of analytic methods adopted from mathematics for solving operational problems. The objective is to provide management with a more logical basis for making sound predictions and decisions.

Ophthalmologist : Specialist in ophthalmology — the branch of medicine which deals with the structure, function, and diseases of the eye.

Ophthalmoscope : An instrument for examining the interior of the eye.

Opioids : Opioids are narcotic analgesics to relieve pain. They are of two types : opium alkaloids (*e.g.* morphine, heroin, codeine), and synthetic narcotics (*e.g.* pethidine, methadone, pentazocine).

Opium : The latex obtained by incision from the unripe capsules of *Papaver somniferum.* Contains about 10% of morphine and has the same function as morphine.

Opportunistic Infections : Infections that affect individuals with HIV infection or inadequacy of the immune system from other causes (*e.g.* herpes, T.B., encephalitis).

Opportunity Loss : The loss incurred because of failure to take the best possible action.

Opposite Event : The event that happens when a given event does not occur.

Optical Disk : In computers, a high capacity and rapid recovery memory device using a laser record and read technique.

Optician : A maker of optical instruments, including spectacles.

Optimal Decision : In a decision analysis, the optimal decision is a decision to select the action that maximizes the decision maker's objective.

Optimal Sample Size : A sample size that yields to minimum total loss.

Optimization : The attainment of the best possible results, *i.e.* the maximization (minimization) of some desirable (undesirable) criterion measure, subject to the constraints imposed on the choice of solutions.

Optimum Feasible Alternative : The alternative among all feasible alternatives that gives the best results or advances the objectives the greatest quantity.

Optometer : An instrument for measuring the refraction of the eye.

Oral Cycle : A 1-month supply of oral contraceptive pills designed to prevent pregnancy within a woman's menstrual cycle.

Oral Contraceptive : Steroid compounds taken by mouth by women to prevent contraception; the "pill".

Orchidectomy : Surgical removal of a testis.

Orchitis : Inflammation of the testicles. It may be a complication of mumps.

Order Effect : A statistically significant difference between treatment conditions due to the order of presentation in a repeated-measures design. Order effects are removed by altering the order of treatments among subjects.

Ordered Array : Simple rearrangement of the individual observations in order of magnitude.

Orderly : A person, usually male, assisting with various routine nursing duties, particularly lifting and moving patients.

Ordinal Measurement : A measurement in which the individual is located in one of a number of mutually exclusive categories that have an inherent logical order.

Ordinal Scale : A classification of cases into a set of ordered classes such that each case is considered equal to greater than, or less than every other case.

Ordinate Axis : The vertical or *Y* axis of a graph, usually used to designate the frequency.

Organic : Pertaining to organs or to living substances.

Organized Medical Staff : A formal organization of physicians and other health care personnel with the delegated authority and responsibility to maintain proper standards of medical care and to plan for continued betterment of that care.

Orgasm : The climax of sexual intercourse.

Ornithosis : A virus infection of man acquired from birds.

Orthodontics : The branch of dentistry concerned with the prevention and treatment of dental irregularities and malocclusion.

Orthogonal Factors : Factors that are not correlated with each other; factors obtained through orthgonal rotations.

Orthogonal Rotation : The operation through which a simple structure is sought under the restriction that factors be orthogonal (or uncorrelated); factors obtained through this rotation are by definition uncorrelated.

Orthopaedics : The branch of surgery concerned with the preservation and restoration of the function of the skeletal system.

Orthopnea : The need to sit upright in order to breathe comfortably, manifested by persons with congestive heart failure.

Osmosis : The passage of a solvent through a membrane from a dilute solution to a more concentrated one.

Ossification : The process of forming bone.

Osteitis : Inflammation of bone.

Osteoarthrosis : A chronic degenerative condition of the joints, usually most marked in the weight-bearing joints.

Osteochondritis : Inflammation of both bone and cartilage.

Osteomalacia : Softening of the bones, with resultant skeletal deformity; associated with lack of vitamin D in adult life.

Osteomyelitis : Inflammation of the bone marrow.

Osteopath : A practitioner of Osteopathy — a medical practice in which manipulation of bones plays a leading part.

Osteoporosis : Increased porousness of bone due to lack of calcium salts in older people.

Otalgia : Earache.

Other Diagnoses : All conditions that coexist at the time of admission, that develop subsequently, or that affect the treatment received and/or length of stay (See also *Principal Diagnosis*).

Otitis Media : Inflammation of the middle ear.

Otoplasty : Plastic surgery for correction of malformed ears.

Otorhinolaryngology : The branch of medicine dealing with diseases of the ear, nose and throat.

Otorrhea : Chronic malodorous discharge from the ear.

Otosclerosis : The form of deafness due to new formation of spongy bone in the middle and internal ear.

Outbreak : A sudden or violent increase in disease activity. A localized epidemic.

Outcome : The end result or effect of care as delivered. Its impact on patients.

Outcome Assessment : The quality of care as judged by the end results of care, such as disability, dysfunction, mortality, morbidity, and satisfaction.

Outcome Variable : The dependent or criterion variable in a study.

Outliers (Outlying Cases) : Those cases falling at either extreme of the bell curve (*e.g.* very short or very long hospital stays). Such cases can have disproportionately strong effects on statistics.

Out-migration : A demographic term meaning exit from a politico-geographic unit (called *emigration* if the unit involved is a country).

Out-of-Scope : A term to describe those reports of vital events which should not be included in a given estimate because they refer to events that took place outside the time period being studied. (See also *In-Scope*)

Outpatient : A patient who receives care without being admitted for inpatient or resident care (*i.e.* clinic, ambulatory, surgery).

Outpatient Clinic : Section without formal beds for treatment and with no staff for patient monitoring.

Outpatient Unit : An outpatient care division that is organized into sections (clinics), the number of which depends on the size and the degree of departmentalization of the medical staff, available facilities, and the needs of the patients for whom it accepts responsibility.

Outpatient Visit : The visit of an outpatient to one or more units or facilities located in or directed by the provider maintaining the outpatient health care services (clinic, physician's office, hospital).

Output : 1. Something that is put out or produced. 2. The process that consists of the delivery of data from a data processing system or from any part of it.

Ovarian Cyst : A sac containing fluid or mucoid material arising in the ovary.

Ovariotomy : The surgical excision of an ovary or of an ovarian tumour.

Overall Confidence Level : The degree of certainty that a group of confidence intervals all include the population parameters they estimate.

Overall Significance Level : An upper bound for the probability of mistakenly rejecting any of a group of null hypotheses when all of the hypotheses are true.

Overall Standard Deviation : The standard deviation for the combined sample with all the observations.

Overdose : The use of any drug in such an amount that acute adverse physical or mental effects are produced.

Overheads : The costs pertaining to general services which do not arise form the operation of a given programme.

Over-population : A condition of excess population; the existence of too many people in a given area, with the result that their standard of living is at a subsistence or near-subsistence level.

Over-the-Counter (OTC) Drugs : Drugs advertised to the customer and sold without prescription; also called *proprietary drugs.*

Ovulation : The process whereby the mature ovum is released from the fully ripened vesicular follicle into the uterine tube.

Oxygenator : A machine for the extracorporeal oxygenation of blood.

Oxygen Therapy : Administration of oxygen—to patients who are having trouble breathing—through the use of an *oxygen tent* or *mask.*

Oxytocin : A hypothalmic hormone stored in the posterior pituitary which stimulates uterine contractions and milk ejection.

Oxyuriasis : Pinworm infection.

Ozena : A chronic disease of mucous membrane of the nose, giving off a very foul-smelling odour or discharge.

P

Pacemaker : In medicine, the sino-atrial node in the right atrium which normally controls the rate of the heart. **Artificial Pacemaker :** A battery which is used to control the rate of the heart when the normal pacemaker is unable to function.

Package : In computers, a set of commercially available programmes designed for a specific use.

Packet : A computer term denoting a short block of data containing information on its source, content and destination which is the unit tansferred in a packet switched network.

Packet Switched Network : A communication network in which packets are transmitted to particular receivers.

Paediatrician : A doctor who specializes in the care of children from the time they are born until they are teenagers.

Paediatrics : The branch of medicine dealing with the diseases and disorders of childhood.

Paedophilia : A sexual preference for children, boys or girls or both, usually of prepubertal or early pubertal age.

Paging : To call over the hospital loudspeaker system. A doctor who is needed to attend a patient can be reached anywhere in the hospital in this manner.

Paired Samples : Samples obtained by pairing subjects to obtain two samples or by measuring something twice for a single sample of subjects. For example, in a clinical trial, pairs of patients may be studied. One member of each pair receives the experimental regimen and the other receives a control regimen. Afterwards both may be tested for any significant difference.

Paired *t* Ratio : Statistical test of the hypothesis of difference between two sample means where the sample selection is not independent.

Paired *t* Test : The statistical method for comparing the difference in a numerical variable observed for two paired (or matched) groups. It also applies to before and after measurements made on the same group of subjects.

Pairwise Disjoint Events : Events such that no two events can happen at the same time.

Palliative : Mitigating, but not curing. A medication that relieves.

Palpation : The method of clinical examination by means of the laying on of hands to establish the size and shape of underlying organs or tumours, the state of the skin, and so forth.

Palpitation : Fluttering. Consciousness of the beating of the heart, usually evoked by unduly rapid, or irregular, action of the heart.

Palsy : Paralysis of any voluntary muscle as a result of some disorder in the nervous system, sometimes accompanied with involuntary tremors.

Pancreatitis : Inflammation of the pancreas.

Pandemic : The term applied to a disease affecting a wide area such as a whole country or continent.

Panel Consensus Method : A method for forecasting in the absence of a relevant data base in which experts within the organization derive a forecast that represents a consensus of the opinions of the experts.

Panel Study : A combination of cross-sectional and cohort methods, in which the investigator conducts a series of cross-sectional studies of the same individuals or study sample. This method permits changes in one variable to be related to changes in other variables.

Papilloma : A benign tumour of surface epithelium, appearing as a warty or papillary overgrowth.

Pap Smear : Papanicolau smear. A procedure for the detection of cancer and precancerous conditions of the female genital tract.

Papule : A small solid elevation on the skin; a solid pimple containing no pus or fluid.

Paracentesis : Tapping or piercing of a body cavity with a trocar and cannula for the purpose of withdrawing fluid.

Paraesthesia : Abnormal cutaneous sensations of numbness, tingling or burning.

Paralysis : Loss of muscular power due to interference such as nerve supply. Palsy.

Paramedical : Related to the medical profession in a supporting or supplementary manner. A paramedical technician has some training in his/her speciality, but not as much as a doctor. Paramedical technicians are often called *allied health professionals.*

Parameters : Values which vary according to the circumstances of their application. Each health problem has a unique set of parameters, that is, plans, tests, and treatments that are individually adapted to that problem.

Parametric Statistics : Statistical tests that require specific distributional assumptions.

Paranoid : A person affected with paranoia (a mental disorder marked by well systematized delusions of grandeur and persecution).

Paraplegia : Paralysis of the lower part of the body and of the lower limbs.

Parapsychology : The study of extra-sensory phenomena.

Parasite : An organism that lives on another at the expense of the latter (or host).

Parasite Density : The collective degree of parasitemia in a population, calculated by the use of either the geometric mean or the weighted average of the individual parasite counts.

Parasitology : The scientific study of parasites.

Paratenic Host : A second, third, or subsequent intermediate host of a parasite, in which the parasite does not undergo any development or replication, but remains, usually encysted, until the paratenic host is ingested by the definitive host of the parasite.

Paratyphoid : An acute infectious disease which resembles typhoid fever but is less severe.

Parenteral : Introduced other than by the mouth (for example, by subcutaneous or intramuscular injection).

Paresis : Partial or temporary paralysis.

Pareto Chart : A bar chart used in quality-control to separate the important problem areas from the less important ones. The bars are drawn in order of decreasing height from left to right.

Parity : The number of live children a woman has borne.

Parkinson's Disease : A progressive disease characterized by muscular stiffness, rhythmic tremor, abnormal gait, and loss of facial expression. Usually a disease of later life.

Paronychia : Pus-producing infection of tissues around the nails, caused by yeasts or bacteria.

Parotitis : Inflammation of the parotid gland.

Paroxysmal : Occurring in, or having the attribution of a paroxysm (a sudden onset or recurrence. A spasm or convulsion).

Parthenogenesis : A sexual reproduction by the development of an unfertilized ovum, seed, or spore.

Partial Correlation : Correlation technique that allows for the ruling out of the possible effects of one or more variables on the relationship among the remaining variables.

Partial Hospitalization : A programme for hospital patients who, for therapeutic purposes on a scheduled basis, regularly use the facilities of the hospital for a substantial number of either daytime or nighttime hours.

Particulate Matter : Particles of solid or liquid matter in the air, including nontoxic materials (soot, dust, and dirt) and toxic materials (lead, asbestos, suspended sulphates and nitrates, etc.).

Parturition : The process of childbirth.

Passage : The transfer of micro-organisms from human to animal host(s) either directly or via laboratory culture.

Passive Smoking : The involuntary inhalation of smoke, usually tobacco smoke, from another person's smoking; known to have a detrimental effect on people in the smoker's immediate environment.

Pasteurization : The method of sterilizing milk by raising it to a temperature of either 72 °C for at least 15 seconds, or 63 to 65 °C for half-an-hour and then cooling immediately.

Patent : Wide open.

Path Analysis : A causal modelling method and correlational procedure, used to test a set of hypothesized cause-and-effect relationships among a series of variables which are logically ordered on the basis of time.

Pathogen : A micro-organism or substance causing disease.

Pathogenicity : The capability of an infectious agent to cause disease in a susceptible host.

Pathology : The science of the study of the causes of disease and the morbid changes they produce in the body.

Patient : A person who is ill or who is undergoing treatment for disease.

Patient Care Audit : An objective, systematic evaluation of the quality of patient care based on pre-established principles.

Patient Compliance : Extent to which patients follow guidance and instructions provided during treatment or on discharge. Specifically, the extent to which they take medicines or self-administer other prescribed treatment.

Patient Data : Information gathered during a patient encounter with a professional health care provider.

Patient Day : See *Inpatient Service Day.*

Patient Monitoring : The use of electronic devices to keep constant watch over a patient's vital signs.

Patient Satisfaction : Extent to which patients express positive attitudes toward specified treatments or to care in general. Often determined by administration of patient satisfaction questionnaires.

Pattern Analysis : A programme to evaluate the effectiveness of medical care evaluation by comparing similar data over time. It is generally directed at the comparison of data regarding particular topics or characteristics.

Payoff Table : In a decision analysis, a two-way table displaying the payoffs, either opportunity losses or profits, for selecting a particular action given that a specific state of nature is in effect.

Pearson *r* : Statistical technique introduced by Karl Pearson for showing the degree of relationship between two variables. The *r* values range from +1.00 (perfect positive correlation) through zero to −1.00 (perfect negative correlation). The farther the Pearson *r* is from zero (in any direction), the stronger is the relationship between the two measurements.

Pediculosis : Infestation with lice.

Pedigree : A diagram showing the ancestral relationships and transmission of genetic traits over several generations of a family.

Peer Review : Technique for appraising quality of care in groups of individuals selected for their similar status and common interests. Can also involve determination of action for quality improvement.

Peer Review Organization (PRO) : U.S. organization which scrutinizes care provided by individual practitioners and health care facilities who wish to treat publicly funded Medicare/Medicaid patients (known earlier as the *Professional Standard Review Organization—PSRO).*

Pellagra : A disease caused by lack of nicotinic acid in association with protein deficiency, and characterized by dermatitis, diarrhoea, and dementia.

Pemphigus : A skin eruption characterized by blebs or bullae.

Pentose : A monosaccharide with only five carbon atoms in the molecule. The most important pentose is ribose.

Perceived Morbidity : The state of ill health as recognized, felt, and reported by the individual and not necessarily identical with clinically observed or scientifically confirmed morbidity.

Percentage : A method of standardizing for size which indicates the frequency of occurrence of a category per 100 cases. A population multiplied by 100.

Percentile : A value on a scale of 100 that indicates the percentage of a distribution that is equal to or below it. For example, 75th percentile for a group of hospitalized patients may be six days, which means that 75% of the patients stayed six days or less.

Percentile Rank : The value that indicates a given percentile. A point at the 90th percentile is said to have a percentile rank of 90.

Per cent Occupancy : See *Bed Occupancy Ratio*.

Percussion : The diagnostic procedure of tapping the surface of the body with a finger or small hammer known as a plessor, to determine the underlying parts.

Percutaneous : Administration through the skin, as by rubbing, injection, etc.

Per Diem : The daily rate for reimbursement of hospital expenditures. It is usually based on the hospital average daily cost and is unlikely to reflect the costs of treating any given case.

Performance Testing : A dry run of the particular computer application to see if the results produced match the specifications laid out in the study phase.

Perfusion : The introduction of fluids into the body by passage through the blood vessels.

Perianal : Situated around the anus.

Pericarditis : Inflammation of the pericardium (the fibroserous sac surrounding the heart).

Perinatal Death : An all-inclusive term referring to both still born infants and neonatal deaths.

Perinatal Mortality Rate : The number of deaths of foetuses weighing at least 500 g (or, when birthweight is unavailable, after 22 completed weeks of gestation), plus the number of early neonatal deaths during a stated year, per 1,000 total births.

Perinatal Period : The perinatal period commences at 22 completed weeks (154 days) of gestation (the time when birth weight is normally 500 g), and ends seven completed days after birth.

Periodontal Disease : Disease of the bony and soft tissues surrounding the teeth.

Peripheral Equipment : In a data processing system, any equipment, distinct from the central processing unit, which may provide the system with outside communication or additional facilities.

Peristalsis : The worm-like movement of the intestine and other tubular organs, characterized by alternate waves of relaxation and contractions.

Peritoneum : The sac of serous membrane that lines the abdominal wall and is reflected over the contained viscera.

Permissible Exposure Limit (PEL) : An occupational health standard to safeguard employees against dangerous chemicals or contaminants in the workplace.

Permutation : Any of the total number of groupings possible within a group.

Pernicious : Vicious, destructive. **Pernicious Anaemia** : A megaloblastic anaemia due to deficiency of vitamin B_{12}.

Personal Hygiene : Those protective measures, primarily within the responsibility of the individual, which promote health and limit the spread of infectious diseases, chiefly those transmitted by direct contact.

Personal Identification : The unique number assigned to each patient within a hospital that distinguishes the patient and his or her hospital record from all others in that institution.

Personality : The ingrained patterns of thought, feeling and behaviour characterizing an individual's unique lifestyle and mode of adaptation, and resulting from constitutional factors, development, and social experience.

Personality Disorder : A variety of conditions and behaviour patterns of clinical significance that tend to be peristent and appear to be the expression of the individual's lifestyle and mode of relating to self and others.

Personal Monitoring Device (PMD) : An instrument attached to a person to measure the exposure of that person to hazardous substance(s).

Personnel Office : The office concerned with hiring and firing employees, and ensuring that working conditions are acceptable.

Personnel Sub-System : A management concept which considers that functional part of a system which provides, through effective development and implementation of its various elements, the human performance necessary in the operation, maintenance, support and control of the system in a specified environment.

Person-Time : A measurement combining persons and time, used as denominator in person-time incidence and mortality rates. It is the sum of individual units of time over which the persons in the study populations have been exposed to the condition of interest.

Pertussis : Whooping-cough.

PERT : *P*rogramme *E*valuation *R*eview *T*echnique. A set of principles, methods and techniques for effective planning of objective-oriented work thereby establishing a sound basis for effective scheduling, costing, controlling, and replanning in the management of programmes.

Pessary : An instrument or appliance for insertion into the vagina to support a prolapsed uterus. A solid body suitably shaped for vaginal administration and containing medicaments intended to act locally.

Pesticide : A substance or agent that is lethal to fungi, insects and the like.

Petechiae : Tiny pinpoint haemorrhages under the skin.

Pethidine (Meperidine) : A synthetic opioid and narcotic analgesic.

Petit Mal : Minor epilepsy. A type of epilepsy in which there are attacks of momentary unconsciousness : distinguished from *grand mal*.

Phagocytosis : The process of ingestion and digestion by cells. The response of phagocytes to invasion by microbes and the like.

Phallus : The embryonic progenitor of the penis in the male and the clitoris in the female. Commonly used now as a synonym for the penis.

Pharmaceutical Drugs : Drugs available from pharmaceutical sources, *i.e.* manufactured by the pharmaceutical industry or made up by a pharmacist.

Pharmaceutical Policy : The system of regulations intended to affect the availability of and demand for pharmaceutical drugs. Synonymous terms are *Drugs Policy* and *Medicines Policy*.

Pharmacist : A dispensing chemist, a chemist and druggist.

Pharmacoepidemiology : The study of the distribution and determinants of drug-related events in a population, and the application of this study to effective drug treatment.

Pharmacokinetics : The study of the rate of drug action, particularly with respect to the absorption, distribution, metabolism and excretion of drugs and metabolites.

Pharmacologist : One who studies the action of drugs.

Pharmacology : The science and study of the action of drugs on the body.

Pharmacy : The science and art of the preparation, combination and dispensing of drugs. The premises where such dispensing is performed.

Pharmacy Committee : Committee responsible for development of policies and practices relating to the selection and distribution of drugs.

Pharyngitis : Inflammation of the pharynx; sore throat.

Phenobarbitone : A widely used barbiturate as a sedative and anticonvulsant.

Phenol : Carbolic acid. A bactericide and an anti-pruritic.

Phenomenon : Any fact, circumstance, or experience that is apparent to the senses and that can be scientifically described or appraised.

Phenotype : The visible traits that characterize the members of a group. See also *Genotype*.

Phenylketonuria : Presence of phenylpyruvate, etc. in the urine. A form of mental deficiency due to the inability of the individual to metabolize phenylalanine as a result of the congenital absence of the enzyme phenylalanine hydroxylase.

Phi Coefficient : Based on chi-square, a measure of the degree of association for nominal data arranged in a 2×2 table.

Phimosis : Elongation and tightening of the foreskin of the penis, preventing retraction over the head of the organ.

Phlebectomy : Surgical excision of a vein or a section of it.

Phlebitis : Inflammation of a vein.

Phlebotomy : "Bloodletting" by cutting into a vein; venesection.

Phlegm : Mucus, particularly that expectorated from the respiratory tract.

Phlegmatic : Dull, sluggish, apathetic, hard to rouse to action.

Phobia : An abnormal, excessive dread or fear.

Phonetics : The science of speech and sound production.

Photophobia : Intolerance of light or morbid fear of light.

Phthisis : Any wasting disease, but usually restricted to the progressive wasting associated with chronic active pulmonary tuberculosis.

Physical Medicine, Physical Therapy, Physiotherapy : Department specializing in rehabilitative services. **Physical Therapy**, utilizes heat, massage, and exercise to rehabilitate muscles, nerves and bones.

Physician : Another name for a doctor of medicine who is trained in the practice of medicine or treating sick people.

Physician Contact : A consultation with a physician in person or by telephone, for examination, diagnosis, treatment, or advice.

Physician Identification : The unique number assigned to each physician, across all hospitals and data systems, that distinguishes the physician from all others in the system.

Physician Referral : The referral of a patient to an inpatient or outpatient hospital facility, for diagnostic or treatment services, by his or her personal physician.

Physician Speciality : Any specific branch of medicine in which a physician may concentrate, *e.g.* psychiatry, endocrinology, plastic surgery.

Physiology : That branch of science that deals with the function of the living body.

Pica : A craving to eat strange foods or unnatural substances – wood, clay, coal, dirt, chalk, etc.

Pie Chart : A circular diagram divided into segments, each representing a category or subset of data. The amount for each category is proportional to the angle subtended at the centre of the circle and hence to the area of the sector.

Pile : Haemorrhoid. A painful swelling of a vein in the region of the anus, often with bleeding.

Pill : A special or ovoid mass containing one or more medicaments.

Pillai Trace : A test statistic used in the multivariate approach to repeated-measures analysis of variance.

Pilonidal : Denoting a growth of hair in a cyst.

Pilot Study : A small-scale study of the methods and procedures to be used on a larger scale if the exercise demonstrates that these methods and procedures can work.

Pinworm : Threadworm. *Enterobius vermicularis.* Sometimes found as a parasite in the human rectum and large intestine.

Pixel : The smallest dot or picture element which can be coded into an electrical signal.

Placebo : An inactive preparation given to control subjects in trials of a similar-appearing active preparation (vaccine, drug, etc.); used to reduce bias in clinical studies.

Placebo Effect : The subjective element introduced by the application of any treatment.

Placenta : The organ on the wall of the uterus through which the foetus receives nourishment and eliminates wastes.

Plague : A bacterial infection caused by *Pasteurella pestis.* **Bubonic Plague,** the common form, characterized by enlargement of the lymphatic nodes (buboes).

Plan : A strategy consisting of a set of steps to achieve goals or objectives.

Planning : The selection of courses of action through a systematic consideration of alternatives in order to attain organizational objectives.

Plantar : Pertaining to the soles of the feet.

Plasma : The fluid portion of the blood, as distinguished from the corpuscles, used for transfusions.

Plasmodium : The genus of the class sporozoa, which includes the causative organisms of malaria.

Plaster : A substance intended for external application, as a support, as a means of applying medicaments, or for the purpose of taking an impression of a part.

Platelet : An oval, colourless blood cell, which is concerned in the process of coagulation (normal range, 250,000 to 500,000 per cubic ml). Thrombocyte.

Platyhelminthes : A phylum which includes flatworms, some of which are parasitic on man.

Platykurtic : A symmetrical curve that is broader (or relatively flat) than a normal curve. This reflects the fact that the scores, are spread more widely than a normal or leptokurtic curve.

Plaque : Tiny patches or unnatural formations on tissues such as on tooth surfaces and on inner arterial walls.

Pleurisy : Inflammation of the pleura (the serous membrane that surrounds the lungs).

Pleurodynia : Excruciatingly sharp pain in the muscles between the ribs.

Plumbism : Lead poisoning.

Pneumococcus : The causative organism of lobar pneumonia. *Diplococcus pneumoniae.*

Pneumoconiosis : Fibrous induration of the lungs due to chronic inhalation of irritant dusts.

Pneumonectomy : Removal of an entire lung.

Pneumonia : Inflammation or infection of the lung; caused by any of a number of agents, such as bacteria, or viruses.

Pneumothorax : The presence of air or gas in the pleural cavity.

Pock : The characteristic pustule of smallpox.

Podiatrist : Chiropodist. One who deals with the treatment of diseases of the hands and feet.

Point-biserial Correlation : A correlational analysis used when one variable is continuous and the other variable is dichotomous.

Point Estimate : The use of a sample value for predicting a single population value. For example, the use of the sample mean for estimating μ is a point estimate.

Point of Intercept (*a*) : In a scatter plot, the point of intercept is the location where the regression line crosses the ordinate, or the value of Y when X is equal to zero.

Poisoning, Alcohol or Drug : A state of major disturbance of consciousness level, vital functions, and behaviour following the administration in excessive dosage (deliberately or accidentally) of a psychoactive substance.

Poisson Distribution : A probability distribution used to model the number of times a rare event occurs. It is a special case of the Binomial Distribution in which the number of individuals involved is very large and the chance of one of the two possible outcomes occurring is very small.

Policy : A basic guide to action that prescribes the boundaries within which activities are to take place.

Poliomyelitis : Inflammation of the grey matter of the spinal cord (caused by polioviruses), accompanied by paralysis of muscles and leading to permanent deformities.

Pollinisis : A state of allergic reaction to inhaled plant pollens (*e.g.* hay fever).

Pollutant : Any substance that renders the atmosphere or water foul or noxious to health.

Pollution : Any undesirable modification of air, water, or food by substance(s) that are toxic or may have adverse effects on health, or that are offensive though not necessarily harmful to health.

Polycythemia : Too many red cells in the blood.

Polydactyly : More than the normal number of five fingers or toes.

Polydipsia : Enormous thirst, characteristic of *diabetes insipidus.*

Polygon : A figure, usually a closed figure, that has more than four sides and angles.

Polyphagia : Voracious eating.

Polyps : Smooth outgrowths or tumours of mucous membranes which line body cavities.

Polyuria : The passage of excessive amounts of urine.

POMR : *P*roblem *O*riented *M*edical *R*ecord. A system of organizing data entries in a patient record by titled and numbered problems that are determined by the clinician in reviewing the patient's direct data, and the data base. Plans for investigation, treatment, and patient education as well as progress recording are all keyed to the problem numbers and titles.

Pooled Standard Deviation : The standard deviation used in the independent-groups *t*-test when the standard deviations in the two groups are equal.

Popliteal : Pertaining to the hind part of the knee joint.

Population : The group of all individuals (usually a very large number) who are the focus of the investigation (for example, all children born to mothers over 35 years of age).

Population at Risk : People who stand a chance of contracting a specified disease (*e.g.* during an epidemic outbreak).

Population Census : The total process of collecting, compiling, and publishing demographic, economic and social data pertaining at a specified time or times, to all persons in a country or delimited territòry.

Population Density : The total number of inhabitants in a country, divided by the surface area.

Population Parameter : A descriptive index whose value refers to the population at large, as opposed to a sample of the population (*e.g.* a population mean or population proportion).

Population Pyramid : Diagram comparing the proportions of males (on left) and females (on right) at every age level.

Population Transfer : Large-scale displacement of people.

Portal Entry : Avenue by which a parasite enters the host.

Positive Correlation : Linear association of increasing values of one variable with increasing values of another variable.

Positively Skewed : Skewed with the tail on the right.

Post-Enumeration Survey (PES) : A special purpose household survey conducted after a main enumeration activity in order to assess the quality of the original enumeration.

Posterior Probability : The conditional probability calculated by using Bayes' Theorem. It is the predictive value of a positive test or a negative test.

Post-facto Research : A type of research that, while not allowing for direct cause-and-effect conclusions, does allow the researcher to make better than chance predictions.

Post-marketing Surveillance : A process implemented after a drug has been licenced for public use, designed to provide use of the drug for a given indication, and information on the occurrence of side effects, adverse reactions, etc.

Post-menopausal : After menopause.

Post-mortem : After death. The examination of a body after death. Necropsy.

Post-neonatal Death : The death of a live-born infant from 28 days to the end of the first year of life.

Post-neonatal Mortality Rate : The number of infant deaths after the first 28 days of life during a stated year per 1,000 live births occurring in the same year.

Postoperative : Occurring in the period after a surgical operation.

Postpartum : After parturition or childbirth.

Postprandial : After a meal; especially after-dinner. Postcibal.

Post-term Neonate : Foetus or newborn with 42 completed weeks or more (294 days or more) of gestation.

Post-test Odds : In diagnostic testing, the odds that a patient has a given disease or condition after a diagnostic procedure is performed and interpreted; similar to the predictive value of a diagnostic test.

Postulate of Parsimony : This stipulates that, given two or more equally compatible models for the given data, the simpler model is believed to be true. In factor analysis, only the model involving the minimum number of common factors is considered appropriate.

Potency : The strength of a particular drug, toxin, or hazard; the ratio of the dose of a standard amount required to elicit a specific response, to the dose of the test agent that elicits the same response.

Potential Years of Life Lost (PYLL) : A measure of the relative impact of various diseases and lethal forces on society. PYLL highlights the loss to society as a result of youthful or early deaths.

Poverty : A condition in which income is insufficient to meet subsistence needs.

Poverty Line : The income or expenditure level below which a minimum, nutritionally adequate diet plus essential non-food requirements are not affordable.

Power : A measure of the sensitivity of a statistical test. The more powerful a test is, the less is the likelihood of committing the beta (Type II) error, *i.e.* accepting the null hypothesis when it should have been rejected.

Power Curve : A function that gives the probabilities of rejecting the null hypothesis for all possible values of the parameters tested.

Power Index : A numerical value used in the calculation of sample size that incorporates a measure of the Type I and Type II error risks that the study planner believes are acceptable.

Pragmatic Study : A study whose aim is to improve health status or health care of a specified population, provide a basis for decisions about health care, or evaluate previous action.

Preadmission Review : Review of necessity for hospitalization prior to admission to determine if it is medically necessary and if the hospital is the appropriate level of care.

Precursor : An early stage in the course of a disease, or a condition or state preceding pathological onset of a disease.

Predicted Score : In linear regression, the score on the criterion that is estimated for subjects with a specific score on the predictor.

Prediction : An estimate of the value of a variable, or the outcome of an event, based on available information regarding related factors.

Predictor : In linear regression, the variable from which criterion scores are estimated; an independent variable.

Pre-eclampsia : A disease of late pregnancy characterized by hypertension, proteinuria and often oedema, which if untreated, progresses to eclampsia.

Pre-existing Condition : See *Comorbidity*.

Pregnancy, Gestation : The state of being with child. **Gestation :** The period from conception to birth.

Pregnancy Termination : The expulsion or extraction of a dead foetus or other products of conception from the mother, or the birth of a live born infant.

Premature Delivery : A baby delivered with time and/or weight factors qualifying it for a premature status.

Prenatal : Before birth.

Prepaid Care : Health programme which offers the patient the opportunity to pay for health care regularly whether it is needed or not, in exchange for which no charge is made when care is provided.

Preposterior Analysis : An analysis that specifies the optimal decision rule based on the possible types of evidence that can be produced by additional information if it is collected.

Presbycusis : Normal diminution of acuteness of hearing that comes with increasing age.

Presbyopia : The impairment of vision which occurs with advancing years.

Prescription : An order for drugs, preparations or appliances, given in relation to a named person by a duly qualified medical practitioner, or registered dentist.

Pre-term Neonate : Foetus or newborn with less than 37 completed weeks (less than 259 days) of gestation and birth weight of less than 2,500 g (up to and including 2,499 g).

Pre-test Odds : In diagnostic testing, the odds that a patient has a given disease or condition before a diagnostic procedure is performed and interpreted; similar to prior probabilities.

Prevalence Rates : 1. **Point Prevalence Rate :** The number of persons with a condition, such as a symptom or pathological lesion, present *at a point in time,* divided by the estimated population at risk; usually expressed per 1,000. 2. **Period Prevalence Rate :** The number of persons with a particular condition (or abnormality) identified over a stated *period of time,* divided by the estimated average population at risk; usually expressed per 1,000 per unit of time.

Preventive Medicine : The application of preventive measures by clinical practitioners in order to promote and maintain health and well-being and prevent disease, disability, and premature death.

Priapism : Abnormal, painful, sustained erection of the penis, unrelated to sexual stimuli.

Prickly Heat : See *Miliaria.*

Primary Diagnosis : The diagnosis chiefly responsible for the major part of the patient's hospital length of stay, as identified by the physician (in some cases, this is a different diagnosis than the principal diagnosis).

Primary Health Care : Essential health care, made accessible to all at a cost the country and community can afford, with methods that are practical, scientifically sound and socially acceptable.

Primary Education : Education at the first level, the main function of which is to provide the basic elements of education, such as elementary schools.

Primary Health Care Approach : The establishment of a health system as described in the Alma-Ata Report, with primary health care as the central function and main focus supported by the rest of the health system.

Primary Prevention : Prevention of the initial occurrence of a disease or other health problems such as low birth weight through such measures as health education, immunization, improvement of the environment and appropriate care of women during pregnancy.

Primary Question : The research question that ties at the heart of an investigation and the answering of which is crucial to the success of an investigation.

Primary Sampling Unit (Cluster) : In multistage sampling, a well delineated area considered to include characteristics found in the entire population.

Primary Variance : Variability of the dependent variable which is assumed to have been produced by the direct action of the independent variable.

Primigravida : A woman who is pregnant for the first time.

Primipara : A woman who has given birth for the first time.

Principal Diagnosis : The diagnosis of the condition after study which is chiefly responsible for occasioning the admission of the patient in the hospital for care.

Principal Procedure : The procedure performed for definitive treatment rather than one performed for diagnostic or exploratory purposes, or one which was necessary to take care of a complication.

Printout : The printed data document from a computer operation. An on-line patient admission system in a hospital may create a printout of the admission information to be used as an identification and summary sheet in the hospital patient record.

Prior Probability : The unconditional probability used in the numerator of Bayes' theorem. It is the prevalence of a disease prior to performing a diagnostic procedure.

Privacy : A right. To declare information confidential is to recognize formally the patient's inherent right to privacy.

Private Consumption : The market value of all goods and services, purchased or received as income in kind by households and non-profit institutions.

Privileged Communication : Any information acquired by a physician or surgeon in attending a patient which was necessary to enable him or her to prescribe or act for the patient and which cannot be revealed in a civil action without the consent of the patient.

Probabilistic Model : A model that incorporates some random element in its formulation as opposed to a deterministic model.

Probability (P) : The statement as to the number of times a specific event can occur out of the total possible number of events. Probability is expressed in decimal form, *i.e.* a probability of 1/20 is written as .05.

Probability of Survival : Chance that somebody alive at a particular age will still be alive at a given older age.

Probability Distribution : A frequency distribution of a random variable, which may be empirical or theoretical (*e.g.* normal, binomial).

Probability Sampling : A sample obtained in a way that ensures that every member of the population has a known, non-zero probability of being included in the sample.

Probability Theory : The branch of mathematics dealing with the purely logical properties of probability. Its theorems underly most statistical methods.

Probability Tree : A visual model to display the outcomes of an experiment in which each successive branch of the tree corresponds to a step necessary to generate the possible outcomes of an experiment.

Proband : The index case or individual who is responsible for the initiation of a genetic study. Propositus.

Problem : An aspect of the patient that disturbs or endangers the patient's health and that requires further attention for diagnosis, treatment, or observation.

Procedural Risk : A professionally recognized risk that a given procedure may induce some functional impairment, injury, morbidity, or even death.

Procedure : A surgical or non-surgical operation, diagnostic procedure, or special treatment assigned by the physician and recorded on the medical record of patients.

Process : Organized series of activities or events which comprise production of goods or delivery of service. In health care, comprises all components of delivery including diagnosis, treatment, aftercare, and health promotion.

Process Assessment : Evaluation based upon what happens in the course of treatment; it considers the professional management of patients.

Process Control : Systems and procedures for ensuring that production and service processes do not vary beyond predetermined limits. Most frequently employed in the manufacturing industry and in areas of health care where material objects are processed or produced (*e.g.* medical laboratories).

Process Control Chart : Chart displaying specified limits of variation with which actual variation (in products or services) can be compared. Excessive variation leads to modification of the process of production or delivery.

Process Indicator : A measure of the extent, efficiency or quality of service performance (*e.g.* proportion of pneumonia cases seen who receive standard case management at health facilities).

Processing, Real Time : The processing of information or data in a sufficiently rapid manner so that the results of the processing are available in time to influence the process being monitored or controlled. Synonymous with *Real Time System*.

Processor : In a computer, a fractional unit that interprets and executes instructions.

Proctitis : Inflammation of membrane of the rectum.

Proctology : That branch of medicine concerned with diseases of the rectum and anus.

Prodromal : Premonitory; early warning signs of an oncoming condition before overt symptoms appear.

Product Moment : The product of moments. The technique by which correlation and trend formulae are derived.

Professional : One who renders a personal service, possesses a specialized body of knowledge, observes ethical principles, maintains high standards and participates in continuing education.

Profile Analysis : Retrospective reviews through which aggregate patient care data are compiled to analyze the pattern of health care services and lengths of stay.

Progeria : Premature aging.

Prognosis : Outlook with regard to the outcome of an illness, *e.g.*, complete recovery, partial recovery, or death.

Programme : An organized aggregate of activities directed towards the attainment of defined objectives and targets, which are progressively more specific than the goals to which they contribute.

Programme Budgeting : The process of making resources available to attain the objectives of programmes. It differs from ordinary budgeting in that the emphasis is on the results to be achieved rather than on unconnected budgetary items.

Programme, Computer : The complete plan for the solution of a problem, more specifically the complete sequence of coded machine instructions and routines necessary to solve a problem.

Programmer Analyst : A professional position in which the capabilities of a computer programmer are combined with some functions of the systems analyst.

Progress : In programming, the carrying out of the component activities of a programme in accordance with the planned schedule.

Progressive Hospital Care : The concept of treating a person only as much as is necessary as an inpatient. Afterwards they take advantage of the hospital's facilities on an outpatient basis.

Prohibition : Policy under which the cultivation, manufacture, and/or sale of a psychoactive drug are forbidden. The term applies to alcohol in general.

Projection : Type of estimate made by a formal deduction from certain stated assumptions.

Prolapse : The sinking down, or falling, of an organ.

Pronatalist : Policy of a government, society, social group, or religion aimed at increasing population growth.

Prophylaxis : Prevention. Preventive treatment.

Proportion : The number of observations with the characteristic of interest divided by the total number of observations; used to summarize counts.

Proportional Allocation : An allocation procedure that partitions the sample size among the strata proportional to the size of the strata when using stratified random sampling.

Proportionate Mortality (Specific Disease) : The proportionate mortality from a specific disease is the number of deaths from the specific disease, divided by the number of deaths from all causes.

Proprietary Hospital : A hospital that is run to make a profit.

Prospective Study : A study (also called a cohort or follow-up study) that follows its subjects forward in time from initial exposure (or non-exposure) to some suspected risk factor, to the eventual disease outcome.

Prostatectomy : Surgical excision of the prostate (a glandular body surrounding the urethra in the male).

Prostatitis : Acute or chronic inflammation of the prostate gland.

Prosthesis : An artificial replacement : *e.g.* an artificial limb.

Prosthodontics : The branch of dentistry that pertains to the replacment of missing teeth and oral structures by artificial devices.

Protected *t*-Test : In analysis of variance, procedures for conducting multiple comparisons between pairs of group means while keeping the experiment-wise error rate at a reasonable level.

Proteinuria : The presence of protein in the urine.

Protocol : A document that rigorously details the objectives of an investigation and how those objectives will be achieved in the investigation.

Prototype : The first full-scale model of a new type or design that exhibits the essential features of the chosen alternative or solution.

Provider : A business entity which furnishes health care to a consumer; it includes a professionally licensed practitioner who is authorized to operate a health care delivery facility.

Provisional Diagnosis : A tentative diagnosis made at the time of patient admission to a health care facility which describes the morbidity of the patient but may not be based on the results of diagnostic tests or procedures.

Proxy Indicator : An indicator used in place of a direct indicator which may be more difficult to measure or compute (*e.g.* school absenteeism may be used as a proxy indicator for general morbidity in school-age children).

Pruritis : Severe itching.

Psittacosis : An epizootic disease of birds which may affect man. The causative organism is a virus.

Psoriasis : A chronic disease of the skin, characterized by elevated lesions in various parts of the body.

Psychedelic : Characterized by freedom from anxiety and by the enjoyment of highly creative, coloured thought patterns.

Psychiatry : The branch of medicine concerned with the study, treatment, and prevention of disorders of the mind.

Psychoactive (Psychotropic) Drug : A substance or drug that, when ingested, affects the mind or mental processes, *e.g.* cognition or affect.

Psychoanalysis : The theories and practice of the Freudian school of psychology.

Psychogenic : Of emotional or mental origin.

Psychology : The branch of science concerned with the working of the mind and mental processes.

Psychoneurosis : An emotional disturbance in which the individual suffers from persisting unwarranted fears and anxieties, lack of self-confidence and general interest in life.

Psychopath : An individual who is suffering from a persistent disorder or disability of mind which results in abnormally aggressive or seriously irresponsible conduct.

Psychosis : Severe mental illness in which the personality is very seriously disorganized and contact with reality is usually impaired. Insanity.

Psychosomatic : Designating a physical disorder of the body originating in the psychic or emotional process of the individual.

Psychotherapy : Treatment of mental disorder by any of various means involving communications between a trained person and the patient and including suggestion, counselling, psychoanalysis, etc.

Pterygium : Growth of the conjunctiva in the corner of the eye nearest the nose, due to a degenerative process caused by long-continued irritation of the tissues.

Ptosis : Drooping of the upper eyelid. Prolapse of any organ.

Puberty : The span of years during which the sex glands become capable of exercising their reproductive functions.

Public Health : A social institution or discipline which endeavours to reduce the amount of disease, premature deaths, and disease produced discomforts and disability in the population.

Public Sector : That part of the economy of a country that comes within the scope of central government, local government authorities and public corporations.

Puerperium : The period succeeding labour, during which the genital organs return to their pre-pregnancy state. The duration is usually 6 – 8 weeks.

Pulse : The rhythmic dilation of an artery produced by ventricular systole.

Pulmonary : Pertaining to, or affecting, the lungs.

Purchaser : Health authority or other organization in a National Health Service which buys care from providers. Implies financial transaction in internal market.

Purgative : A drug for causing evacuation of the bowels. Cathartic.

Purposive Selection : The deliberate selection of a sample because it is believed to be representative of the target population.

Purpura : A condition characterized by the occurrence of purple spots in the skin, due to extravasation of blood in the skin.

Purulent : Concerned with, or containing, pus.

Pus : The liquid product of inflammation, containing leucocytes, dead or dying micro-organisms and cellular debris.

Pustula, Pustule : A small elevation of the skin containing pus.

Putrefaction : The decomposition of living matter, particularly protein, usually by bacteria assisted by enzymatic action.

***P*-Value :** The probability of observing a result as extreme as, or more extreme than, the one actually observed from chance alone (*i.e.* if the null hypothesis is true).

Pyelocystitis : Inflammation of the pelvis of the kidney and the bladder.

Pyelogram : An X-ray picture of a kidney visualized with a radio-opaque medium.

Pyelonephritis : Inflammation of the kidney, including the pelvis.

Pyemia : Pus in the blood.

Pyogenic : Producing pus. Pyopoietic.

Pyorrhoea : A discharge of pus. **Pyorrhoea alveolaris,** periodontal disease with a purulent discharge.

Pyrexia : A fever, or febrile condition.

Pyrogen : A fever-producing substance .

Pyrogenic : Fever inducing.

Pyrosis : Heartburn.

Pyuria : Pus in the urine.

Q

Q fever : A rickettsial disease resembling pneumonia, often mild and unrecognized.

q.i.d. : Four times a day.

QALY : *Q*uality *A*djusted *L*ife *Y*ears. A measure of the outcome of actions in terms in their health impact. If an action gives a person an extra year of healthy life expectancy, that counts as one QALY. Death is rated as 0.

Quack : An untrained person who practices medicine fraudulently.

Quadripara : A woman who has given birth to four viable children. Para IV.

Quadriplegia : Paralysis of all four limbs. Total paralysis of the body from the neck down.

Quadruplet : One of four children born at one birth.

Qualitative Data : Data that does not have a quantitative scale (for example eye colour, sex, nationality, etc.).

Qualitative Variable : A variable defined by its characteristics. For example, an independent variable might have three levels that differ in the type of drug used for treating a disorder.

Quality : A characteristic (physical or non-physical, individual or typical) that constitutes the basic nature of a thing or is one of its distinguishing features (*e.g.* the *quality* of health care in a country).

Quality Assessment (Quality Appraisal) : The measurement of the level of quality at some point in time with no effort to change or improve the level of care.

Quality Assurance : Activities performed to determine the extent to which a programme (such as health care) fulfils certain values and standards, and to assure changes in practice that will fulfil the highest level of values.

Quality Assurance Mechanism : Retrospective review programmes by the organized medical staff. It assumes the quality of care as compared to locally or internally developed standards and verifies that the standards or exceptions are met, that deficiencies are corrected, and that the original problem is reassessed on a planned programme basis.

Quality Control : The management process of establishing standards or product output specification and the techniques for ensuring that the standard or output is monitored and held in stable balance.

Quality Documentation : Records used in the practice of quality assurance. Alternatively, records describing quality systems and procedures.

Quality Management : Process of continuous planning, implementation and evaluation of quality assurance structures, systems, procedures and activities. Implies emphasis on human factors including motivation and development of quality culture.

Quality of Care : A level of performance or accomplishment that characterizes the health care provided (in terms of manpower, facilities, diagnostic or therapeutic procedures, outcome, utilization, and levels of patient satisfaction).

Quality System : Arrangements for exchange of information and liaison between components of quality structures. The way structures are expected to function.

Quantify : In analysis, to translate observed physical relationships into analogous mathematical relationships.

Quantiles : Divisions of a distribution into equal, ordered sub-groups. *Deciles* are tenths; *quartiles,* quarters; *quintiles,* fifths, *terciles,* thirds; and *centiles,* hundredths.

Quantitative Analysis : Descriptive statistics; a basic means of describing and understanding the population served by the health care system; includes demographic information, health status information, and utilization of services.

Quantitative Data : Data with a numerical scale (for example, ages, weights, etc.).

Quantitative Variable : A variable defined by its amount. For example, an independent variable might have three levels that differ in drug dosage.

Quantity Index : An index that measures the change in the value of a set of goods attributed only to changes in quantities with prices being held constant.

Quarantine : Isolation of individuals who have been in contact with highly infectious diseases. The period (originally 40 days) during which an arriving vessel suspected of carrying contagious disease is detained in ports in strict isolation.

Quartan : Occurring every fourth day, counting both days of occurrence : said of a fever (*e.g.* Quartan malaria, a type of malaria in which the paroxysms occur every fourth day).

Quartiles : Divisions of a distribution representing quarters; the first quartile representing the 25th percentile, the second quartile the 50th percentile, and the third quartile the 75th percentile.

Quartimax : A criterion for obtaining an orthogonal rotation; the emphasis is on simplifying the rows of the factor pattern matrix.

Quartimin : A criterion for obtaining an oblique rotation, the oblique counter-part of the quartimax rotation, requires the introduction of reference axes.

Queasiness : Feeling of nausea.

Quellung : The capsular swelling that occurs in bacteria when mixed with specific antibody.

Questionnaire : A predetermined set of questions used to collect data—clinical data, social status, occupational groups, etc. A self-completed survey instrument.

Quetelet Body Mass Index : Weight divided by the second power of height multiplied by 100, an anthropometric index proposed in 1835 and still widely used to quantify the relation between height and weight in the diagnostic assessment of eating disorders.

Queue : A line of people, such as patients in a primary health care centre, usually waiting.

Quick : A tender, vital part, as the bed of a fingernail.

Quickening : The first foetal movements felt by the mother, usually in the 4th or 5th month of pregnancy.

Quiescent : Inactive, at rest.

Quinine : An alkaloid from cinchona, used as an anti-malarial, especially against *plasmodium falciparum;* also used for its analgesic, oxytocic and antipyretic properties.

Quinsy : Inflammation of the throat due to peritonsillar abscess.

Quintan : Recurring every fifth day, as a fever.

Quintipara : A woman who has given birth to five viable offspring Para V.

Quintuplet : One of five children born at the same birth.

Quivering : Shaking or trembling.

Quota : In demography, maximum number of immigrants of a given type legally permitted to enter a country (often based on nationality).

Quota Sampling : A method used for selecting a representative sample which is based on drawing subjects in proportion to their existing percentages in the population (for example, if 35% of a certain population is composed of women, then 35% of the sample must be made up of women).

Quotidian : Recurring every day (*e.g. quotidian malaria,* vivax malaria in which the febrile paroxysms occur daily).

Quotient : The result obtained by dividing one number by another. **Intelligence Quotient** : A number indicating a person's level of intelligence; it is the mental age multiplied by 100 and divided by the chronological age.

R

Rabies : A viral infection of the brain of certain animals, particularly dogs and wolves, which is transmitted to man by the bite of an infected animal and causes hydrophobia.

Race : A population that differs from others in the relative frequency of some gene or genes. Any group of people having the same ancestry.

Radex : The hypothetical size of the birth cohort in a life table, commonly 1,000 or 100,000.

Radiation Sickness : Sickness produced by over exposure to radiation, as from X-rays or atomic explosions, and characterized by nausea, diarrhoea, bleeding, loss of hair, and increased susceptibility to infection.

Radiculitis : Inflammation of a spinal nerve root.

Radioactivity : The property of emitting radiation by the spontaneous disintegration of certain nuclides or their nuclei.

Radiograph : The X-ray photo.

Radiologist : A physician specializing in the use of X-rays.

Radiology : The science of X-rays and their use for diagnostic purposes in medicine.

Radioscopy : Examination of the image thrown by X-rays on a fluorescent screen.

Radiosensitivity : The capacity of tissues to react with different degrees of intensity to radiation.

Radiotherapy : The use of ionizing radiations in the treatment of disease.

Rales : Abnormal sounds from the lungs or air passageways, heard over the chest.

Random Access Memory : Memory which is used for temporary storage of programmes and data within a computer and is erased when the power is shut off.

Random : Governed by chance, not completely determined by other factors. As opposed to deterministic.

Random Clinical Trial : An experimental study in which subjects are randomly assigned to treatment groups.

Random Error (or Variation) : The variation in a sample that can be expected to occur by chance.

Random Factors : Unsystematic sources of variation. Individual difference variables and experimental errors are random factors.

Randomization : The process of assigning subjects to different treatments (or *vice versa*) by using random numbers or a chance governed mechanism.

Randomized Block Design : An experimental design whereby treatments are randomly assigned within a set of blocks to eliminate bias.

Random Misclassification : Imprecise categorization of a person as exposed or non-exposed, or as diseased or non-diseased; it can only alter the rate ratio toward 1.0.

Random Number : A number selected from a population in such a way that it has the same probability of occurring as does every other number in the population.

Random Number Table : A table of numbers constructed in a way that ensures that (1) each of the numbers 0 through 9 has probability 1/10 of occurring in any position in the table, and (2) the occurrence of any number in one part of the table is independent of the occurrence of any number in any other part of the table.

Random Sample : Sample selected in such a way that every element or individual in the entire population has an equal chance of being chosen.

Range (R) : Difference between highest and lowest values in the set of values; it describes the entire width of the distribution.

Rank Correlation Coefficient : A correlation coefficient for ranked (rather than numerical magnitude) observations.

Rank of a Matrix : The number of linearly independent columns or rows of a matrix; the order of the largest square sub-matrix whose determinant is not zero.

Rank-order Scale : A scale for observations arranged according to their size, from lowest to highest or *vice versa*.

Ranks : A set of observations arranged according to their size, from lowest to highest or *vice versa*.

Rank-sum Test : A non-parametric procedure for testing hypotheses about the difference in location between two populations; used when data are in the form of ranks.

Rash : An eruption of red spots on the skin, usually temporary.

Rate : A rate is a measure of some event, disease, or condition in relation to a unit of population, along with some specification of time; usually multiplied by a constant, such as 1000, 100,000 etc.

Rate Difference : One rate minus another rate with the same dimensions; the units correspond to those of the rates.

Rate of Growth : The rate of natural increase combined with the plus or minus factor of net immigration or net emigration.

Rate of Natural Increase : A measure of annual population growth based on the difference between the birth rate and the death rate per 1,000 population.

Rate Ratio : One rate divided by another rate with the same dimensions; a unitless measure of association.

Ratio : A part divided by another part, *i.e.* the quotient of two numbers. It is the number of observations with the characteristic of interest, divided by the number without the characteristic. All rates are ratios, but not all ratios are rates.

Ratio Data : Data that provide information regarding the order of numbers, the difference between numbers, and also an absolute zero point; permits comparisons, such as *A* being three times *B*, or one-half of *B*.

Ratio Estimation : An estimation procedure based on the relationship between two variables y and x that have been measured on the same set of sampled elements.

Ratio Scale : A scale of measurement that has all the characteristics of an interval scale, plus a meaningful zero point.

Ratio to Moving Average Method : A method for measuring seasonal variations by means of monthly or quarterly indexes.

Raw Score : A quantitative score obtained in a study which is not subjected to any statistical transformations; also called an *original score.*

Re-admission : Subsequent admissions of a patient to a hospital or other health care institution for treatment.

Real Birth Cohort : A group of births occurring at the same time.

Real Cost : Cost expressed in terms which have been adjusted for inflation which enables comparisons to be made between expenditures.

Real Time Processing : A form of interactive processing in which the computer system records each change immediately and updates all the necessary files, etc. immediately. In health information, a computerized on-line appointment system could be real time; intensive care computers that monitor patient heart functions, breathing, etc. are real-time systems.

Reason for Encounter : The patient's complaints and symptoms reflecting his/her own perception of his/her needs provided verbally or in writing by the patient at the point of entry into the health care system, or that patient's own words recorded by an intermediary or provider at that time.

Record Control : That part of medical record retention and retrieval that provides (1) defined limits on retrieval of the data by particular users, and (2) methods to communicate continually the current location of a record.

Record Destruction Programme : A plan that includes a time schedule and facility for routinely eliminating selected medical records from the files.

Record Linkage : The process of connecting one individual's medical records, even though they were developed at different times and in different places and combining them into one file by means of a common identifier.

Recovery Room : The room in which a patient recovers from an operation or recovers from the delivery of an infant.

Recrudescence : The recurrence of symptoms after a temporary abatement.

Rectangular Distribution : A distribution wherein each score occurs with the same frequency.

Rectocoele : A bulging of the rectum through the rear wall of the vagina.

Recurrent Expenditure : Current operating expenditure. Covers items that recur year after year such as staff salary, cost of goods and services, replacement of equipment, and the maintenance of buildings and equipment.

Redundancy : The existence of more than one means for accomplishing a given function.

Reference Axes : These refer to the axes that are orthogonal to the primary factors; they are introduced to simplify oblique rotation.

Referenced Diagnostic Service : Provision of laboratory resources by a hospital to physicians of a given community. Specimens such as blood or tissue, may be sent to the lab for examination. The hospital does it as a service to the community.

Reference Population : The standard against which a population that is being studied can be compared.

Referred Outpatient : An outpatient who is provided special diagnostic or therapeutic service of the hospital for diagnosis or treatment on an ambulatory basis. The responsibility for medical care remains with the referring physician.

Referred Pain : Pain that doesn't originate where it hurts.

Reflex : Involuntary response to a stimulus.

Reforestation : The establishment of plantations for industrial and non-industrial uses; it does not include regeneration of old tree crops.

Refraction : In ophthalmology, the measurement and correction by lenses, of defects of the eye which prevent light waves from being brought to sharp focus exactly on the retina.

Refractometer : An instrument for measuring the refractive power of the eye and other translucent substances.

Refugee : Person who migrates of his own volition but in response to powerful pressure to leave.

Regimen : A prescribed course of treatment.

Registered Nurse (RN) : Nurse who has completed a two-to four-year course at an approved nursing school and has been licensed to practice after passing an official examination.

Registered Record Administrator (RRA) : A medical records professional who has achieved a specified educational level and has successfully completed a national qualifying examination.

Registration Data : Data derived from certificates of vital events; births, deaths, marriages, divorces; and notifiable diseases.

Registry : A synopsized listing of data that categorizes a larger group of data. Registries are usually constructed to provide meaningful data for important disease conditions within a society (*e.g.* cancer registry).

Regression : A set of statistical procedures that allows a researcher to use the value of one variable to predict the value of another variable.

Regression Analysis : The process of fitting a regression equation to a set of data by using the method of least squares; also includes the various statistical tests and estimates associated with the use of the fitted equation.

Regression Equation : An equation that describes the linear relationship between a dependent variable and one or more independent variable.

Regression Line : The single straight line that lies closest to all the points in a scatter plot.

Regular Frequency Distribution : A listing of every score value, from the lowest to the highest, together with the number of times that each score was obtained (its frequency).

Regurgitation : Effortless casting of food from the stomach soon after eating; "spitting up" of food.

Rehabilitation : As applied to disability, the combined and coordinated use of medical, social, educational, and vocational measures for training or re-training the individual to the highest possible level of functional ability.

Reiter's Syndrome : A form of arthritis with inflammation of the mucous membrane of the eyes and of the urethra.

Rejection Region : In the theory of hypothesis testing the set of values such that if the test statistic assumes one of these values, the null hypothesis is rejected.

Relapse : Return of a disease after apparent recovery.

Relapsing Fever : Episodes of fever which subside spontaneously, then recur.

Relative Bias : A measure of the relative error of a measurement process attributable to systematic error, *i.e.* the bias of a process divided by the true value of the quantity being measured.

Relative Cyclical Residual : The percentage deviation from trend because of cyclical and irregular factors.

Relative Frequency : The ratio of the number of observations (elements) in a class (subset) to the total number of observations constituting a population (universe or set).

Relative Risk : The ratio of the incidence of a given disease in exposed or at risk persons to the incidence of the disease in unexposed persons; calculated in cohort or prospective studies.

Relative Survival Rate : The ratio of the observed survival rate for the patient group to the expected survival rate for persons in the general population similar to the patient group with respect to age, sex, race, and calendar year of observation.

Release : A written instrument by which some claim or interest is surrendered to another person (for example, the release that a potential surgical patient signs before the operation).

Reliability : The extent to which a measuring instrument measures consistently.

Reliable Data : Information obtained by means of a well-defined objective method for measurement which involves all or a representative sample of patients and practitioners.

Relvariance : A shortened form of the term "relative variance", *i.e.* the variance of an estimate divided by the square of its expected value. The relvariance of an estimate is also equal to the coefficient of variation squared.

Remission : A temporary diminution or abatement of signs and symptoms during an illness.

Renal : Pertaining to the kidney.

Renal Dialysis : Procedure used by patients who have lost the use of their kidney. Their kidney function must be replaced two or three times a week by a renal dialysis machine.

Renal Insufficiency : Incapacity of the kidneys to filter toxins adequately from the blood.

Repeated-measures Design : A study design in which subjects are measured at more than one point in time; also called a *split-plot design* in ANOVA.

Repellent : A chemical applied to the skin or clothing or other places to discourage (1) arthropods from alighting on and attacking an individual, or (2) other agents, such as helminth larvae, from penetrating the skin.

Replacement Level Fertility : The level of fertility at which a cohort of women are having only enough daughters to replece themselves in the population; equal to a net reproduction rate of 1.00.

Replication : The execution of an experiment or survey more than once so as to confirm the findings, increase precision, and obtain a closer estimation of sampling error.

Report of a Disease : An official report notifying an appropriate authority of the occurrence of a specified communicable or other disease in man or in animals. Reports may also list suspect cases of diseases of particular public health importance, ordinarily those requiring epidemiological investigation.

Representative Sample : A sample that reflects the characteristics of the entire population. Random sampling is assumed to result in representative samples.

Reproductive Isolation : Absence of interbreeding between populations.

Reproductive Pattern : Described in terms of parental age and spacing and total number of children.

Reproductive Wastage : Loss of life from fertilization of ovum to fifth year of age.

Reprogramming : Revising a programme on the basis of evaluation if it is found that the programme is not acceptable to the people for whom it is intended, is not proceeding according to plan, or is inefficient.

Requirement Analysis : The first stage in the development of a computer application in which the system is described in terms of the problem to be solved and the benefits to be derived from its solution.

Research : A quest for new knowledge pertinent to an identified area of interest (a problem), through application of the scientific process.

Research and Development (R&D) : Basic and applied research in the sciences and engineering, and the design of prototypes and development of processes. Excludes routine product testing, market research, sales promotion, service, and other non-technological activities.

Research Hypothesis : A statement (prediction) about the expected outcome of a study.

Resection : Surgical removal of part of the body.

Reservoir (mechanism) : Mechanism for perpetuating agent species.

Reservoir (of Infectious Agents) : Any person, animal, plant or substance in which an infectious agent normally lives and multiplies, on which it depends primarily for survival, and where it reproduces itself in such manner that it can be transmitted to a susceptible host.

Residence : The place in which a person resides long enough to qualify for certain rights, privileges, etc.

Residency Programme : An accredited programme whereby a hospital sponsors post-graduate medical education for physicians in training.

Resident Day : See *Inpatient Day*.

Residential Care Facility : A facility that provides custodial care to persons who, because of their physical, mental, or emotional condition, are not able to live independently.

Resident Service Days : See *Inpatient Service Days*.

Residual : The difference between the predicted value and the actual value of the outcome (dependent) variable in regression.

Residual Plot : In regression analysis, any plot of the residuals used to check regression assumptions.

Residual Urine : Significant amount of urine left in the bladder after urination.

Resistance : The sum total of body mechanisms which interpose barriers in the progress of invasion or multiplication of infectious agents or to damage by their toxic products.

Resolving Power : The capacity of a system to distinguish between truly distinct things that are close together.

Resonance : The sound produced on percussion over a part that can vibrate freely, *e.g.* the lungs.

Resources : The means to meet objectives : the supply of manpower, materials, money, equipment and such.

Resources Allocation : The process of distributing available material and personnel among a set of users.

Resource Management : The efficient and effective management of resources by implementing rational use of manpower, knowledge, facilities, and funds in order to achieve the intended purposes with the greatest effect for the least outlay.

Respirator : An apparatus for maintaining respiration, as in patients with paralysed muscles of respiration.

Response Rate : The number of completed or returned survey instruments (questionnaires, interviews, etc.) divided by the total number of persons who would have been surveyed if all had participated, usually expressed as a percentage.

Restriction of Range : Low variability, caused by the way in which the samples were defined, that will underestimate the correlation between that variable and other variables.

Resuscitation : Artificial respiration applied to a person threatened with death by asphyxia.

Retching : Ineffective movements of vomiting.

Retention/Retrieval Manual : A written manual that describes the planning, implementation, and control of a system that safeguards the physical and information characteristics of medical or health data for future use.

Reticulation : The determination of boundaries of census areas, units, and other sub-divisions in the country.

Retina : The inner nervous coat of the eye, which is specially adapted for the reception of light stimuli.

Retinal Detachment : Separation of the light-receiving layer of the back of the eye from its underlying layer.

Retinitis Pigmentosa : Hereditary degeneration and atrophy of the retina.

Retinoblastoma : A malignant tumour of the retina.

Retinopathy : Degenerative disease of the retina.

Retrobulbar : Behind the eyeball.

Retroflexion : Condition of being bent backward.

Retrospective Study : An hypothesis-testing study that collects information about past events by direct enquiry from respondents. This, and other data, are then usually related to the distribution of disease in the respondents.

Retroversion : A backward-tilted position of an organ, as a retroverted uterus.

Review : Process of retrospective quality appraisal. Can also involve determination of quality action. Also reconsideration of appropriateness of any aspects of quality assurance or quality management.

Rhesus Factor (Rh Factor) : A group of antigens (observed first in the blood of Rhesus monkeys), determined by heredity and usually present in human red blood cells, which may cause haemolytic reactions during pregnancy or after transfusion of blood containing this factor into someone lacking it. Individuals who have this factor are Rh positive; those who do not have it are Rh negative.

Rheumatism : A generic term used to describe pain of unknown origin affecting the connective and muscular tissues and joints.

Rheumatology : The study of rheumatic diseases.

Rhinitis : Inflammation of the nasal mucous membrane.

Rhinoplasty : Plastic repair of the nose.

Rhinovirus : From *rhino,* meaning nose; large group of viruses, antigenically distinct (over 60 serotypes), but similar in small size, chemistry (RNA), and ability to cause common cold in man.

Ribose : One of the pentose sugars found in nucleotides.

Rickets : A disease, principally of childhood, characterized by various deformities of bone resulting from softening of the bone due to lack of vitamin D.

Rickettsia(e) : Microbial agent(s) appearing like small bacteria and multiplying by simple fission, but only within a living host cell.

Rigor Mortis : The gradual stiffening of the muscle tissue that occurs after death.

Ringworm : Any of various contagious skin diseases caused by three related fungi and characterized by itching and the formation of ring shaped, discoloured patches covered with scales or vesicles.

Risk : Conditional expected loss in a normal-form decision analysis; the probability of an unfavourable outcome.

Risk Approach : The approach consisting of identifying and devoting more care to individuals or groups who, for biological, environmental or socio-economic reasons, are at special risk of having their health impaired, of contracting a specific disease, or of having inadequate attention paid to their health problems.

Risk Benefit Analysis : The process of analyzing and comparing on a single scale the expected positive (benefits) and negative (risks, costs) results of an action, or lack of an action. The result of a risk benefit analysis is called the *Risk Benefit Ratio.*

Risk Factor : A term used to designate a characteristic that is more prevalent among subjects who develop a given disease or outcome than among subjects who do not.

Risk Management : The steps taken to alter, *i.e.* reduce the levels of risk to which an individual or a population is subject.

Road Accident Rate : The number of injured persons in a geographical area during a time period, divided by the estimated population at risk, expressed per 1,000 persons per unit of time.

Robust Statistical Test : A statistical test that gives fairly accurate results even if the underlying assumptions are not met.

ROC Curve : *R*eceiver *O*perating *C*haracteristic curve. In diagnostic testing, a plot of the true-positives on the *Y* axis *versus* the false-positive on the *X* axis; used to evaluate the properties of a diagnostic test.

Rodenticide : A chemical substance used for the destruction of rats and other rodents, generally through ingestion.

Roent (*r*) : A quantitative unit of X-radiation, used in calculating intensity of exposure.

ROM : Abbreviation for "Read only memory". Contains the instructions which start up when power in the computer is turned on.

Root Canal : A small channel in the root of a tooth, continuous with the pulp chamber above it.

Roseola : Any rose-coloured eruption of the skin.

Roughage : The insoluble indigestible material in food, which promotes peristaltic action.

Rounds : Visits made to patients by doctors and nurses at periodic intervals to check on their condition.

Roundworm : A species *(Ascaris lumbricoides)* of nematode worms, living as parasites, especially in the intestines of man and other mammals.

Routine Health Service Records : Records of certain measurements usually taken by health services personnel (*e.g.* birth weight, height, weight), or information as to activities carried out by the health sector (*e.g.* coverage of various kinds, immunization, and treatment of common diseases).

Row Per cent : In a cross tabulation, the result of dividing a cell frequency by the number of cases in the row. Row per cents sum to 100 per cent for each row of a cross-tabulation.

Roy's Largest Root : A test statistic used in the multivariate approach to repeated-measures analysis of variance.

Rubella : German measles. A mild infectious disease, due to a virus, with a characteristic rash.

Rubeola : Measles. Preventable by measles vaccine.

Rubric : Section or chapter heading; used in epidemiology with reference to groups of diseases, *e.g.* as in the *International Classification of Diseases (ICD).*

Run : In a series of observations of attributes the occurrence of an uninterrupted series of the same attribute is called a run.

Runs Test : A test in terms of sequences of identical occurrences that are followed and preceded by different occurrences or by none at all.

Rupture : A break in continuity. Hernia.

Ruptured Disk : Protrusion of the pulpy, cushioning pad between vertebrae through a rent in sorrounding ligament.

S

Saccharin : A sweetening agent and substitute for sugar; also used intravenously as a test for the determination of circulation time.

Sadism : The form of sexual perversion in which pleasure is derived from inflicting cruelty on another.

Safe Water Access : The percentage of population with reasonable access to safe water supply, including treated surface water or untreated but contaminated water such as that from springs, sanitary wells and protected boreholes.

Sago : A starch derived mainly from pith of the sago palms, and used as a foodstuff.

Saline : Salty, containing sodium chloride. **Physiological Saline :** An isotonic salt solution for temporarily maintaining living cells.

Salmonella : Gram negative, non-sporing bacilli; the causative organism of typhoid and paratyphoid fevers; also responsible for outbreaks of food poisoning.

Salpingitis : Inflammation of a uterine tube.

Sample: A smaller number of individuals taken from some population (for the purpose of generalizing to the entire population from which it was taken). The data collected by a researcher.

Sampling Distribution : Distribution made up of measures taken on successive random samples. Two important sampling distributions are the distribution of means and the distribution of differences.

Sampling Error : The expected difference between a measure of the sample and a measure of the population ($X - \mu$), based on chance and chance alone.

Sampling Fraction : The proportion of the population that will be included in the study sample.

Sampling Frame : An available list or other source of sampling units that is the best available representation of the population to be studied.

Sample Space : Outcomes of an experiment; may be discrete and finite, discrete and infinite, or continuous (finite).

Sampling Units : The individual entities that form the focus of a survey. These are often individual people but might be other entities such as individual hospitals, depending on the objectives of the survey.

Sanatorium : An establishment for the treatment of sick individuals, more particularly those requiring prolonged treatment (*e.g.* for TB.).

Sanitation : The science of maintaining a healthy environment.

Sanitation Access : The percentage of the population with reasonable access to sanitary means of excreta and waste disposal, including outdoor latrines and composting.

Sarcoidosis : A non-contagious disease of unknown cause, somewhat resembling tuberculosis.

Sarcoma : A form of cancer arising mainly from connective tissue.

Satyriasis : Excssive and uncontrollable sexual desire in the male.

Scab : The crust that forms on superficial injured areas.

Scabies : A highly contagious, itching infestation of the skin with *Sarcoptes scabiei.*

Scald : The burn caused by hot liquid or vapour.

Scale of Measurement : The nature of the assumptions one makes about the properties of a variable; in particular, whether that variable meets the definition of nominal, ordinal, or interval measurement.

Scalpel : A pointed knife with a convex edge.

Scanning : The operation of looking over a group of objects to find any that may be generating a particular or unique type of information.

Scar : The mark left by a healed wound, ulcer, or breech of tissue.

Scatter Plot : A two-dimensional graph that shows how the values of one variable are related to the values of another variable.

Scenario : A work picture of a fixed sequence of events in a defined environment.

Scheffe's Procedure : A multiple-comparison method for comparing means following a significant F test in analysis of variance. It is the most conservative multiple-comparison method.

Schistosomiasis : (Bilharzia). A parasitic disease of the tropics caused by the free-swimming forms of a blood fluke.

Schizophrenia : A psychosis characterized by disturbance in reality relationships and disintegration in the personality.

Sciatica : Pain in the distribution of the sciatic nerve.

Scleroderma : "Hidebound skin"; a connective tissue disease of unknown cause.

Sclerosis : Hardening of the tissue, especially by overgrowth of fibrous tissue.

SCM : *S*ociety for *C*omputer *M*edicine; an association which promotes the use of computers in medicine.

Scoliosis : Sidewise curvature of the spine.

Scotoma : A dark spot, blind, or partially blind area in the field of vision, indicating some pathological change in optic nerve or retina.

Screening : The identification of unrecognized disease or defect by the application of tests, examination, or other procedures which can be applied rapidly. Screening tests sort out apparently well persons who probably have a disease from those who do not. A screening test is not intended to be diagnostic.

Scrofula : Tuberculosis of lymph gland of the neck.

Scurvy : A deficiency disease due to lack of ascorbic acid (Vitamin C) and characterized by extravasation of blood to various parts of the body, particularly the skin and gums.

Seasickness : Nausea and/or vomiting induced by the movement of a ship at sea.

Seasonal Effect : The rises and falls in a time series, which always occur at a particular time of the year because of changes in the seasons.

Seasonal Index : An index measuring the seasonal effect of a particular month (when using monthly data) or quarter (when using quarterly data).

Seasonal Migrant : Person who moves temporarily at certain seasons of the year.

Seasonal Variation : Change in physiological status or in disease occurrence that conforms to a regular seasonal pattern.

Sebaceous Cyst : A skin tumour produced by obstruction of the outlet of an oil-secreting gland.

Seborrhoea : A disturbance of the skin caused by overaction of the sebaceous glands.

Secondary Attack Rate : The proportion of contacts who get a communicable disease as a consequence of contact with a case. It is a measure of contagiousness and is useful in evaluating control measures.

Secondary Education : Education at the second level, based on at least four years of previous instruction at the first (or primary) level and providing general or specialized instruction, or both.

Secondary Health Care : Specialized care provided at district or provincial hospital level by trained staff in such areas as radiographic diagnosis, general surgery, care of women with complications of pregnancy or childbirth, and diagnosis and treatment of uncommon or severe disease.

Secondary Prevention : Preventive activities that arrest or retard existing disease through early detection and appropriate treatment or to reduce the occurrence of relapses and the establishment of rehabilitative measures.

Secondary Question : A research question that, while interesting and potentially informative, does not form the central focus of an investigation. It is usually intended to supplement the issues in the *primary question*.

Secondary Storage : Storage or memory which is not located in the central processor of the computer but is in peripheral media such as tapes, disks, diskettes, etc.

Secondary Variance : Variability of the dependent variable that is not under experimental control but is instead a result of confounding variables. Holding secondary variance to a minimum helps to ensure a high degree of internal validity.

Secular Trend Analysis : A method, using correlational techniques, for predicting linear trends across time. Historical data are used to forecast results based on the assumption that the past trend will continue.

Security : In computer terminology, the establishment and application of safeguards to protect data, software, and computer hardware from accidental or malicious modification, destruction or disclosure.

Sedative : Any of a group of central nervous system depressants with the capacity of relieving anxiety and inducing calmness and sleep.

Sedimentation Rate : The rate at which red blood cells settle out of a prepared specimen of blood under laboratory conditions.

Segment : A small geographic area used as a cluster, often as an ultimate cluster.

Seizure : A sudden attack of transient abnormality of motor, sensory, or psychological nature associated with transitory cerebral dysfunction.

Self-care : Largely unorganized health activities and health-related decision-making carried out by individuals, families, neighbours, friends and workmates (includes maintenance of health, prevention of disease, and self-applied treatment and follow-up care after contact with the health services).

Self-care Patient : A patient who must continue regular treatments at the outpatient facilities but who does not need much assistance from the medical staff

Self-destructive Behaviour : A collective term for acts entailing injury, or the risk of injury, to the individual concerned, such as uncontrolled drinking, or carrying out suicidal acts.

Self-inflicted Injuries : The injurious effect of suicide and attempted suicide. This includes injuries resulting from self-destructive acts carried out without the intention of dying.

Self-limited : A disease that comes to an end all by itself in a limited time.

Self-reliance : In primary health care the initiative of individuals in assuming responsibility for their own health development, adopting measures that are understood to them, knowing their own strengths and resources, and knowing when to turn to others for support and cooperation.

Self-sufficiency : In primary health care, the practice or tendency of individuals to depend solely on their own strengths and resources in looking after their health care needs.

Semantics : The study of the meaning of words and symbols.

Semen : The thick whitish fluid carrying the spermatozoa.

Semi-Interquartile Range (SIQR) : The interquartile range divided by two.

Seminoma : A tumour of the testes.

Semi-Private Room : A hospital room with two patients.

Senile : Pertaining to old age. Weak in mind and body.

Sensitivity : Ability of a technique to differentiate poor, fair, and good care.

Sensitization : The rendering of an individual, or bacteria, sensitive to a drug, protein or some other substance. Anaphylaxis.

Sentinal Health Events : Instances of particularly poor quality or recurring quality problems in public health which trigger subsequent investigation and quality action (*e.g.* emphasis on sanitation after the 1994 outbreak of plague in certain parts of India).

Separation : When an inpatient leaves hospital to return home, transfers to another institution, or dies.

Separation Diagnosis : The final diagnosis made at, or following, the patient's separation. (The diagnosis made on admission is usually a provisional one.)

Separation Rate : The number of separations per 1,000 total population per year.

Separation Summary : A summary written, or dictated, by a doctor about the case, setting out the essential facts from the record.

Sepsis : The condition characterized by the presence of micro-organism(s).

Septal Defects : Abnormal openings between chambers of the heart, allowing blood to "leak" from one side of the heart to the other.

Septicaemia : The condition characterized by the presence of micro-organisms in the blood stream.

Septuplet : One of seven offspring of a single gestation.

Sequel(a) : A morbid consequence of a disease (plural : sequelae).

Seroepidemiology : Epidemiological study on activity based on the decision on serological testing of characteristic change in the serum level of specific antibodies in order to detect infections and carrier states.

Serology : The study of serum, with particular reference to immunity reactions.

Serum Sickness : A manifestation of delayed hypersensitivity to long-persisting anti-serum of non-human origin (*e.g.* diphtheria or tetanus autotoxin or rabies anti-serum produced in horses); typically begins 10-12 days after inoculation and may be very crippling.

Service Classification : Classification of services provided by the medical staff in terms of functionally autonomous units (departments, divisions, wards) at a given hospital.

Service Industry : Industry in which the primary aim is the effective execution of a series of interactions between people, *i.e.* in which one group of people does things for, to, or with, other groups.

Services : See *Health Care Services*.

Service (or Care) Unit : A group of patients who have related diagnoses and/or kinds of treatment; a group of inpatient beds designated for a single speciality of the medical staff.

Sex : The sum of those differences that distinguish male from female.

Sex Chromosome Abnormality : A disorder of function that is associated with a partial or complete absence of a sex chromosome or with extra sex chromosomes, *e.g.* Klinefelter's syndrome (males with XXY sex chromosomes).

Sex Ratio : Number of males per 100 females.

Sex-specific Death Rate : The ratio of the total number of deaths in a specific sex group in a year, divided by the mid-year population of the same sex group.

Sextigravida : A woman who is pregnant for the sixth time.

Sextipara : A woman who has given birth to six children in the same number of labours.

Sextuplet : One of six children resulting from one pregnancy.

Sexual Assault : Use of physical force or threat of using physical force to compel a person to engage in a sexual act against their will, whether or not the act is completed.

Sexual Counselling : Guidance, support, or education of an individual who presents with problems or questions concerning sexual relationships.

Shift : Period of duty, usually eight hours long; since hospital care must be provided continuously, each day is divided into three shifts.

Shigellosis : An infection with a member of the genus *Shigella,* the causative organism of bacillary dysentery.

Shingles : *Herpes zoster.* An acute virus disease with eruption of blisters on the skin along the course of a nerve.

Shock : A condition in which the vital capacity is profoundly lowered, often as a result of severe injury, and characterized by cold clammy skin, pallor, rapid pulse, and low blood pressure.

Short-stay Patients : Inpatient stays that are 48 hours or less. Also includes outpatients who stay a short time, usually 24 hours or less.

Short-stay Surgery : See *Ambulatory Surgery*.

Sibling : A brother or sister. Any of two or more offspring of the same parents.

Sick Baby : A baby delivered with medical complications, other than those relating to premature status.

Sickle Cell Anaemia : An hereditary abnormality of haemoglobin.

Side Effect : An effect produced by a drug, or some other form of therapy in addition to the derived or expected effect.

Siderosis : A form of pneumoconiosis; chronic lung inflammation due to long inhalation of dusts containing minute particles of iron.

Sight : Vision (the power or range of seeing). **Long Sight**, hypermetropia, **Near Sight**, myopia.

Significant Procedure : A procedure that is surgical in nature, or carries a procedural risk, or carries an anaesthetic risk, or requires specialized training.

Sign Test : A non-parametric test used to analyze paired data and test hypotheses about population medians or population median differences. The test is based on counting the direction (or sign) of each within-pair difference.

Silicosis : The form of pneumoconiosis due to the inhalation of silica-containing dusts.

Simple Frequency Distribution : Scores arranged from highest to lowest, with the frequency of occurrence of each score indicated by a column beside the scores.

Simple Random Sample : A random sampling method that ensures that every member of the population has the same chance of being included in the sample. A table of random numbers is usually employed to select this type of sample. (Also known as EPSEM sample—"equal probability of selection method").

Simulation : The representation of physical systems and phenomena by computers, models or other equipment. The model or computer representation is manipulated to imitate significant aspects of a situation.

Single Blind Experiment : An experiment in which the experimental subjects cannot distinguish the experimental conditions.

Sinus : A hollow, cavity or channel. A fistula. **Sinusitis**, inflammation of a sinus.

Sitz Bath : Application of wet heat or relieve pain, congestion, spasm, etc., in the pelvic area, by sitting in a tub of warm water which covers only the hips and buttocks.

Size of Completed Family : Number of children in a family whose mother has completed the childbearing period.

Skeleton : The bony framework of the body.

Skewed Distribution : A distribution with some extremely low scores (negatively skewed, skewed to the left) or some extremely high scores (positively skewed, skewed to the right), resulting in a frequency polygon with a pronounced tail in one direction.

Skilled Nursing Facility : An institution with an organized professional staff and permanent facilities, including inpatient beds that provides continuous nursing and other health-related, psychosocial, and personal services to patients who are not in an acute phase of illness but who primarily require continued care on an inpatient basis.

Sling : A piece of material, or a bandage for the suspension of a part—usually the arm.

Slippage : The effective loss of registration reports after they have been prepared by the registrar, but prior to their inclusion in the tabulated vital statistics.

Slipped Disk : See *Ruptured Disk*.

Slope : The angle of a straight line. In linear regression, the change in the regression line for a unit increase in X variable.

Slough : A mass of dead tissue cast off from or contained in living tissue.

Slow Virus : Agent causing degenerative (neurological) diseases characterized by a long incubation period and a prolonged, slowly progressive course (*e.g.* multiple sclerosis, kuru, some cases of AIDS).

Small Upper-arm Circumference : Circumference less than the value corresponding to the 5th percentile of the frequency distribution for well-nourished children.

Smears : Secretions or blood spread on a glass slide for examination under a microscope.

Smegma : The sebum, with a characteristic odour, secreted by the external genitalia.

Smoothing : Processing of averaging in a general way to reduce random fluctuations to a negligible level.

Snare : A wire loop used to remove polyps or small pedunculated tumors.

Snellen Chart : The familiar eye test chart consisting of block letters in diminishing sizes.

Snuffles : The noisy respiration in children induced by persistent nasal discharge interfering with breathing.

Social Class : A stratum of society composed of individuals and families of equal standing.

Social Cost : The total cost to society of any form of economic activity such as the impairment of the health of employees, or air population due to factory chimneys.

Social Drift : Downward social class morbidity as a result of impaired health, often due to mental disorders.

Social Medicine : The practice of medicine concerned with health and disease as a function of group living (*i.e.* health of people in relation to their behaviour in social groups) and involves care of the patient as a member of a family and community.

Social Protection : Provision of social welfare in the areas of health, pensions, unemployment benefits and other income support schemes.

Social Structure : The way groups are organized in a society, and the way the relationship between these groups is defined.

Social Worker : See *Medical Social Worker*.

Software : Computer programmes, procedures, rules and any associated documentation concerned with the operation of a data processing system.

Solid State : The electronic components that convey or control electrons within solid materials, *e.g.* transistors, germanium diodes, and magnetic cores. Thus vacuum and gas tubes are not included.

Somatic : Pertaining to the body.

Somnambulism : Sleep-walking (a state of altered consciousness in which phenomena of sleep and wakefulness are combined *Somnolence* : Sleepiness. *Somnolent* : Sleepy.

Sore : An ulcer. **Bed Sore**, decubitus ulcer; **Cold Sore** : *herpes labialis.* Hard Sore; syphilitic chancre.

Sorter : A machine which puts items of information into a particular order, *e.g.* it will determine whether A is greater than, equal to, or less than B, and sort or order accordingly.

Soundex System : A phonetic filing system that uses a combination of letters and code numbers to designate patient names.

Source Document : Document on which data are originally recorded (hand-written or typed) and from which data elements are extracted for input into a computerized data system.

Source of Infection : The person, animal, object, or substance from which an infectious agent passes to a host.

South-North Gap : A set of national, regional and other estimates in which all figures for developing countries are expressed in relation to the corresponding average figures for all the industrial countries, indexed to equal 100.

Spa : A health resort with mineral springs.

Spasm : A sudden, involuntary muscular contraction.

Spasmolytic : Checking spasms. An agent that relieves spasm.

Spastic : Related to spasm. An individual affected by spasticity.

Spatula : A flat, knife-like instrument used to spread plasters and ointments, and also for depressing the tongue.

Spay : To sterilize (a female animal) by removing the ovaries.

Spearman ρ (rho) : Correlation coefficient devised by C.E. Spearman for use with rank-ordered data (*i.e.* data that have been ranked or ordered with respect to the presence of a given characteristic).

Special Care Unit : A medical care unit in which there is appropriate equipment and a concentration of physicians, nurses, and others who have special skills and experience to provide optimal medical care for critically ill patients, or continuous care of patients in special diagnostic categories.

Specific : Of a specified or particular kind. An age-specific rate is a rate for a particular age group, such as "15-24".

Specification Limits : The upper and lower specification limits are the largest and smallest values that a quality characteristic can have and still be considered acceptable for use.

Specific Fertility Rate : A measure of live births in a specific group. Often refers to births to women in specified age groups, in which case it is called an age-specific rate.

Specificity : The proportion of time that a diagnostic test is negative in patients who do not have the disease or condition. A specific test has a low false-positive rate.

Specific Rate : A rate that pertains to a specific group or segment of the observations (examples are age-specific mortality rate and cause-specific mortality rate).

Spectacles : Framed or mounted lenses worn to assist vision. Eye-glasses.

Speculum : An instrument for dilating an orifice to allow for examination of the passage or cavity beyond.

Speech Therapy : A set of behaviourial techniques and procedures designed originally for the correction of defects of vocalization and articulation, such as stuttering.

Spell of Sickness : An episode of sickness with a well-defined onset and termination; often defined by the duration of absence from work or school.

Spermatocoele : A swelling of the scrotum caused by cystic dilation (fluid-filled sac) of the sperm-conducting tubules of the testicle.

Spermatocide : An agent that kills spermatozoa.

Spermatozoa : The mature male term cells.

Sphincter : An annular muscle that surrounds an orifice and keeps it closed.

Sphygmomanometer : An instrument for measuring the arterial blood pressure.

Spica : A figure-of-eight bandage.

Spina Bifida : Developmental defect of the spine in which part of the central lamina of one or more vertebrae are missing with varying degrees of protrusion of the spinal cord and its meninges.

Spinal Tap : Withdrawal of spinal fluid through a needle; used in the diagnosis of diseases such as meningitis, polio, etc.

Spine : The vertebral column. A short, sharp projection.

Spirit : An alcoholic solution of a volatile substance. Any distilled liquid.

Spirometer : An instrument for measuring the capacity of the lungs.

Spleen Rate : A term used in malaria epidemiology to define the frequency of enlarged spleens detected on survey of a population in which malaria is prevalent; used to summarize the severity of malaria endemicity.

Splenomegaly : Enlargement of the spleen.

Split-unit Experiment : An experiment (also known as a split-plot, repeated-measures, or nested experiment) in which one of the main effects involves between-subjects comparisons while another involves comparisons within the same subject.

Spondylitis : Arthritis of the spine.

Spondylosis : A degenerative lesion of the spine leading to ankylosis.

Sporadic : Scattered. Occasional. Not epidemic.

Spot Map : Map showing the geographic location of people with a specific attribute for the investigation of a localized outbreak of disease.

Spotting : A slight show of blood in the vaginal discharge at times other than menstruation.

Sprain : Injury, usually of a joint, without dislocation, and resulting in tearing or rupture of ligaments with accompanying effusion.

Spreadsheet : A computer programme which is based on the use of tables whose entries can be text, numbers, or formulae relating to other locations in the table.

Sprue : A disease of uncertain origin, due to intestinal malabsorption, and characterized by dyspepsia, glossitis, fatty stools, and loss of weight.

SPSS, SPSS/PC : A statistical software package (*S*tatistical *P*ackage for *S*ocial *S*ciences). *SPSS* is a trademark of *SPSS* Inc. *(SPSS/PC* is the same package for personal computers).

Spud : A flattened, bevelled surgical blade. An instrument used for removing foreign bodies, as from the cornea.

Spur : An outgrowth, usually of bone.

Spurious Relationship : A non-causal relationship between two variables that exists only because of the common influence of a third variable. The spurious relationship disappears if the third variable is held constant.

Sputum : Material from the respiratory passages which is ejected by means of expectoration.

Squint : Strabismus. Being cross-eyed.

Stable Population : Group having constant age-specific birth and death rates and therefore an unchanging age-sex distribution and a population pyramid of fixed shape.

Stain : A dye used in histology and microbiology. A mark or discolouration. To discolour or colour.

Stammering : A disturbance of speech characterized by hesitancy due to difficulty in pronouncing certain syllables, and resulting in their being repeated over and over again. Stuttering.

Standard : Specification of expected or desirable measurable attributes of a product or service. Can be more or less specific than related term criterion.

Standard Deviation : A measure of variability that indicates how far *all* scores in a distribution vary from the mean (denoted by σ in the population and *s* or *sd* in the sample). It is the square root of the variance. It can be used with the mean to describe the distribution of observations (in a normal distribution, the mean plus and minus one standard deviation marks approximately the middle 68% of the scores).

Standard Error of the Difference : An estimate of the standard deviation of the distribution of differences based on the standard deviations of two random samples.

Standard Error of the Mean : An estimate of the standard deviation of the sampling distribution of means based on the standard deviation of a single random sample.

Standard Error of the Proportion : An estimate of the standard deviation of the sampling distribution of proportions obtained in a single random sample.

Standard (or Adjusted) Birth Rate : Specific birth rates applied to some standard age distribution.

Standardized (or Adjusted) Death Rate : Specific death rates applied to some standard population (India, 1990; USA, 1985, etc.).

Standard Marriage Rate : Age- and sex-specific marriage rates applied to a standard population.

Standardized Mortality Ratio : The ratio of the number of deaths observed in the study group to the number of deaths "expected" in the study group under the set of rates for the control population.

Standardized Proportional Mortality Ratio : The ratio of two mortality proportions, expressed as a percentage, usually adjusted for age and/or time differences between the two groups being compared.

Standardizing : Expressing the difference between two values in terms of standard deviations rather than the original units of measurement. Standardized values are often denoted by the letter *z*.

Standard Score : A raw score expressed in standard deviation units. A *z* score and a *T* score are examples of standard scores.

Standard Stillbirth Rate : The number of stillborn infants with a birth weight of at least 1,000 grams per 1,000 births (both live and stillborn).

Staphylococcus : Gram-positive cocci growing in clusters, responsible for a range of infections.

Stasis : Stagnation. The slowing down or stoppage of flow of a fluid.

State of the Art : The current level of sophistication of a developing technology, as of computer science.

States of Nature : In a decision analysis the states of nature are the uncertain events over which the decision maker has no control.

Stationary Population : Group having constant and equal birth and death rates, no migration, and a fixed total size.

Statistic : Any measure that is obtained from a sample as opposed to the entire population. The range (or the mean or the standard deviation) of a set of sample scores is a statistic.

Statistical Artifact : An incorrect conclusion caused by errors in the collection or statistical analysis of data.

Statistical Contamination : The effect of an unrecognized independent variable that works either in the same or the opposite direction to an independent variable under study.

Statistical Controls : The correlation of raw data by statistical methods to make allowance for the existence of biases that could not be controlled in the experimental design.

Statistical Display : A graphic arrangement of statistical information, for example, tables, charts, graphic illustrations, and computer plots.

Statistical Error : Any error in sampling or in the analysis of data, such as using the wrong tests or misinterpreting their outcomes.

Statistical Hypothesis : A numerical statement of the potential outcome of a study.

Statistical Inference : The drawing of conclusions about populations from the statistical analysis of sample data.

Statistical Prediction : Making a prediction, diagnosis, etc., not by intuition but by incorporating the relevant knowledge into a rigorous and explicit framework, and wherever appropriate, using statistical techniques.

Statistically Significant : A term used to indicate that the results of a study are not simply a matter of chance. A statistically significant test leads to rejection of the null hypothesis (*i.e.* the independent variable has indeed had an effect on the dependent variable) and generally interpreted as a result that would occur by chance; *e.g.* 1 time in 20, with a *P*-value less than (<) or equal .05.

Statistical Universe (Population) : The total collection of items that fall within the scope of a statistical investigation.

Statistics : The branch of applied mathematics that deals with the collection, analysis, and interpretation of data, and makes inferences about populations from samples.

Statute of Limitations : A law limiting the period of time during which an action must be brought; the legal requirement regarding retention time periods for various business and medical documents.

Steatorrhea : Stools containing large amounts of undigested fats.

Stem and Leaf Display : A graphical display (similar to both a frequency table and a histogram) for numerical data. In this each observation is divided into a stem value and a leaf value. The stem defines a set of classes, and the number of leaves within a stem defines the frequency with which the values in that class occur.

Stenosis : Constriction or narrowing of a channel, duct, or opening.

Step Chart : Illustration of patterns of motion often used in place of a line chart.

Stepwise Regression : In multiple regression, a sequential method of selecting the variables to be included in the prediction equation.

Stereogram (Isometric Chart) : A graph or chart that displays more than two variables in a manner that appears three-dimensional to the eye.

Sterilization : The process of rendering an individual infertile, or incapable of producing progeny. The destruction of all micro-organisms, usually through the use of heat. Items that have been sterilized are said to be *sterile.*

Sterility : Complete inability to reproduce, either temporary or permanent.

Sterilizer : An apparatus for the destruction of micro-organisms in the process of rendering material sterile.

Steroid : One of a group of substances which have a wide range of biological activities. They include the sex hormones, the hormones of the adrenal cortex, and the bile acids.

Stethoscope : An instrument for listening to sounds produced in the body, particularly those from the heart and lungs.

Stillbirth Rate : The number of stillbirths plus deaths in the first week of life in a geographical area during a time period, divided by the total number of live plus stillbirths, expressed per 1,000 total births per year.

Stillborn Infant : A foetus, irrespective of its gestational age, that after complete expulsion or extraction, shows no evidence of life, *i.e.* heartbeats or respiration.

Still's Disease : A disease of children, like rheumatoid arthritis, affecting many different joints.

Stigma : A mark or blemish. A peculiarity of a given condition which is diagnostic.

Sting : The acute burning sensation produced by the bite of an insect or snake or contact with a poisonous plant, or by some other toxic substance. The organ that produces a sting.

Stitch : A sharp pain, usually at the left costal margin, and often evoked by exercise. A suture.

Stochastic Process : The statistical concept underlying the prediction of the condition of an element of a larger group when the probable average condition of the larger group is known.

Stomatitis : Inflammation of the mucous membrane of the mouth.

Stool : An evacuation of the bowels. Stools, faeces.

Strabismus : The condition in which the visual axes assume a position relative to each other different from that conforming to physiological conditions. Squint.

Straight Line Correlation : Either a positive or negative correlation, so that the points in a scatter diagram tend to form a straight line through the centre of the graph.

Strangulation : Asphyxiation by means of compression of the air passages. Contraction of a part resulting in arrest of the circulation: *e.g.* as may occur in a hernia.

Strategy : The science· of planning, directing and managing an operation.

Stratification : A sampling scheme in which independent sampling plans are used in different, well-defined sub-divisions (or strata) of the population.

Stratified (or Quota) Sampling : Selecting a sample that directly reflects the population characteristics. If it is known that 45% of the population is composed of males, and if it is assumed that gender is a relevant research variable, then the sample must contain 45% of male subjects.

Streptococcus : Gram-positive spherical bacteria, arranged in pairs or chains of varying lengths; responsible for a variety of infections.

Stress : Mental or physical tension. The sum of all non-specific biological phenomena elicited by adverse external influences, including damage and defence.

Stretcher : A sheet of canvas slung between two poles, each with two handles, for the transport of the injured, sick or wounded.

Stricture : Narrowing of a duct, passage or orifice.

Stridor : The harsh, high-pitched respiratory sound produced characteristically by partial laryngeal obstruction.

Stroke : A general term referring to a medical condition often involving paralysis and frequently caused by a blood clot.

Structural Assessment : A judgement as to whether the care is being provided under conditions that lead to the provision of good care. These include such items as the number, mix, and qualifications of the staff, the manner in which the staff is organized and governed, space, equipment, and other physical facilities, and financial arrangements.

Structure : The arrangement of organic units or parts in a whole. The arrangement of constituent parts of a body : the manner of organization.

Student *t* Distribution : A bell-shaped distribution of t values; has a mean of 0; used for making inferences about a population mean when the population variance σ is unknown and the sample size n is small. See also *t-Test*.

Stupor : A state of lowered consciousness. Reduced responsiveness.

Stye : A suppurative inflammation of one of the hair follicles of the eyelids.

Stylet : A fine probe, particularly one used to keep the lumen of a needle or catheter patent. Stilet.

Styptic : Astringent. A local application that arrests haemorrhage.

Subclinical (Silent, Inapparent) Infection : Infection resulting in no clinically evident disease.

Subcutaneous : Beneath the skin, as a hypodermic injection.

Subjective : Influenced by the thoughts of the subject, or researcher. Not unbiased and objective.

Subjective Probability : The degree of belief or confidence placed in the occurrence of an event.

Subject Variable : A characteristic of a subject that is fixed at the time of the experiment and not manipulated by the experimenter. Examples of these variables are age, sex, height, weight, and personality traits.

Subluxation : Partial or incomplete dislocation, sprain.

Substance Use Disorder : Any mental or behavioural disorder resulting from the use of one or more psycho-active substances such as alcohol, opioids, sedatives or hypnotics, cocaine, caffeine, tobacco, etc.

Substernal : Underneath the breastbone.

Sub-system : A series or group of components that perform one or more operations of a more complex system.

Suckle : To nurse at the breast.

Sucrose : A disaccharide present in certain plants such as sugar-cane, beet, etc.

Sudorific : Sweat-inducing.

Sufficiency : A sufficient estimator is an estimator that utilizes all the sample information available.

Suicide : The act of taking one's own life. One who kills himself/herself.

Sum of Squares (SS) : A measure of the total amount of variation present in a set of data. It is obtained by summing the squared deviation between each individual result and the mean, and hence is measured in squared units.

Summary Indices : Values summarizing a set of observations.

Sunburn : The effect of the sun's rays on the skin, ranging from tanning to redness and severe dermatitis.

Sunstroke : A form of heatstroke due to over-exposure and severe dermatitis.

Supine : In the state of supination. Lying on the back, face upwards.

Support System : A composite of equipment, skills, and techniques that is capable of performing a clearly defined function in support of a mission.

Suppository : A solid body suitably shaped for rectal administration, and usually containing medicaments.

Suppression of Zero : A term used to describe a misleading graph that does not have a break (a jagged line) in the *Y*-axis to indicate that part of the scale is missing.

Suppuration : The formation of pus.

Surgeon : A doctor who specializes in surgery.

Surgery : (1) The treatment of disease, injury, etc. by manual or instrumental operation. (2) The operating room of a surgeon or hospital.

Surgical Operation : One or more surgical procedures performed at one time for one patient via a common approach or for a common purpose. See also *Surgical Procedure.*

Surgical Procedure : Any single separate systematic process upon or within the body which can be complete in itself, normally performed by a physician or dentist to restore disunited or deficient parts, to remove diseased or injured tissues, to extract foreign matter, to assist in obstetrical delivery, or to aid in diagnosis.

Surrogate : A substitute. A person who takes the place of another in someone's affective existence (*e.g.* a *surrogate* mother).

Surveillance of Disease : Continuing scrutiny of all aspects of occurrence and spread of a disease that are pertinent to effective control. *Serological Surveillance* identifies patterns of current and past infection using serological tests.

Survey : An observational study that generally has a cross-sectional design; a commonly used design to collect opinions.

Survival Analysis : The statistical method for analyzing survival data when there are censored observations.

Survival Curve : A curve that starts at 100% of the study population and shows the percentage of the population still surviving at successive times for as long as information is available.

Susceptible : A person or animal presumably not possessing sufficient resistance against a particular pathogenic agent to prevent contracting infection or disease if or when exposed to the agent.

Suspect Case : A person whose medical history and symptoms suggest that he or she may have or be developing some communicable disease.

Suspension : A dispersion of solid particles throughout a liquid medium. Temporary cessation. A method of treatment, either by fixation of an organ. or by traction.

Suture : The material by which the two edges of a wound or incision are kept in apposition. The process of uniting edges of a wound or incision.

Swab : An absorbent pad for mopping up cavities or wounds, or for applying medications locally. A sterilized swab on the end of a stick or wire for taking specimens, as from the tonsils, for bacteriological examinations.

Swelling : A prominence. An enlargement.

Swing Beds : Hospital-based acute care beds that may be used flexibly to serve as long-term care beds.

Sycosis : Inflammatory disease of the hair follicles, especially of the beard.

Symbiosis : The biological association of two or more species to their mutual benefit.

Symmetric Distribution : A distribution whose two halves are mirror images of each other, *i.e.* has the same shape on both sides of the mean. The mean, median, and mode are all equal.

Symptom : A manifestation of disease as felt and described by the patient, as opposed to a sign which is a manifestation of disease apparent to the observer.

Synchronous : Pertaining to two or more processes that depend upon the occurrence of a specific event such as a common timing signal.

Syncope : Sudden transient loss of consciousness due to an inadequate supply of blood to the brain.

Syndactyly : Webbing or fusion of the fingers and/or toes.

Syndrome : A collection of symptoms and signs that occur together so often as to provide a recognizable clinical entity.

Synergy : A situation in which the combined effect of two or more factors is greater than the sum of their solitary effects.

Synovial Fluid : The clear viscid fluid, which lubricates the movement of tendons and joints.

Synthetic Birth Cohort : An artificial birth cohort, composed of a cross-sectional sample of the population.

Syphilis : An infectious venereal disease caused by *Treponema pallidum.*

Syringe : An instrument for injecting fluids into the body.

Syrup : A concentrated aqueous solution of sucrose, or other sugars, to which medicaments or flavourings may be added.

System : An integrated relationship of man, equipment and methods appropriately organized to accomplish defined tasks.

Systematic Sampling : A method of selecting a sample by a systematic method as opposed to random sampling, such as selecting each tenth name from a list of patients or by sampling every third resident in every other block in an area sample.

Systemic Disease : One which affects the body as a whole, not limited to a particular part.

Systems Analysis : A problem-solving method for an overall, thorough analysis of an activity to determine the most appropriate method for accomplishing it. It is directed to knowledge and processes required for planning and implementing computer-based systems in health and patient information handling.

Systems Effectiveness : The probability that the system can successfully meet an operational demand within a given time when operated under specified conditions.

Systems Engineering : The application of scientific and engineering knowledge to the planning, design, construction and evaluation of man-machine systems and components.

Systole : The period of blood-pumping contraction of the heart.

T

Table of Random Numbers : A table constructed so that each entry is equally likely to be any five-digit number from 00,000 to 99,999. The table of random numbers is used in selecting a random sample.

Tablet : A compact product containing a medicament or a mixture of medicaments in a moulded or compressed form.

Taboo : A ritual prohibition against a specific behaviour or contact with an object or person, usually punishable by supernatural means.

Tachycardia : Abnormally rapid heart rate.

Tachypnoea : Very rapid breathing.

Taenia, Taeniasis, Taenicide : A genus of tapeworms mostly parasitic on men and animals (*e.g. Taenia solium, Taenia saginata*). **Taeniasis**, refers to infestation with tapeworms and a **taenicide** is a drug or measure that kills tapeworms.

Tail Probability : A probability calculated from an area in the tail or tails (ends) of a distribution.

Talipes : Foot deformity; clubfoot.

Tampon, Tamponade : A pack or plug made of cotton or some comparable material and used as a plug, *e.g.* in the nose or vagina. **Tamponade** refers to the insertion of a tampon.

Tan : The brownish colouration of the skin produced by exposure to sun, wind, or artificial ultraviolet light.

Tape, Magnetic : A tape with a magnetic surface on which data can be stored by selective polarization of portions of the surface.

Tapeworm : A ribbon-like flatworm which may invade the intenstines of consumers of undercooked beef, fish, or pork.

Tapping : Paracentesis. The removal of fluid from a cavity by means of a trocar and cannula. A series of sudden slight blows in massage.

Target : An intermediate result towards the objective that a programme seeks to achieve (*e.g.* the target of immunizing 80% of children against polio by 1998 with a view to immunizing all of them by the year 2000).

Target Matrix : A matrix of coefficients used as a target in rotation; an initial factor solution may be rotated in such a way that the resulting factor loadings resemble the target matrix maximally.

Target Population : The collection of individuals, items, measurements, etc., about which the investigator wants to make inferences or wishes to generalize.

Tartar : A deposition on the teeth of the organic constituents of saliva, along with calcium and magnesium salts and food particles.

Task Analysis : An analytical process employed to determine the specific behaviour required of human components in a man-machine system. It involves determining on a time base the detailed performance required of a man and machine, the nature and extent of their interactions, and the effects of environmental conditions and malfunctions.

Tattooing : Insertion of permanent colours into the skin, through punctures, as by a needle.

Taxonomy of Diseases : The orderly classification of diseases into appropriate categories on the basis of relationships among them, with the application of names.

Tchebycheff's Rule : A method for setting bounds on probability statements.

***t*-Distribution :** A symmetric (bell-shaped) distribution of *t*-values (also called the student *t* distribution) with mean zero and a standard deviation larger than that for the normal distribution for small sample sizes. As *n* increases, the *t* distribution approaches the normal distribution.

Technology : The translation into practical use of the results of scientific research.

Technology Transfer : In public health, the process of the application of scientific discoveries, and of methods, procedures, techniques and equipment that will promote health and socio-economic development.

Telecommunications : The transmission and reception of messages over a distance, *e.g.* using radio, fax, telephone lines.

Telematics : The use of computer-based information processing in telecommunications.

Telemedicine : The use of telematics to transmit medical data.

Teleprocessing : Data processing through the use of a combination of data processors, or computers, and telecommunications facilities.

Teletext : A computer-based information retrieval system which uses screen messages broadcast by television or provided interactively through a cable system.

Telex : A process of digital telecommunication of alphanumeric characters.

Temporary Staff : Physicians or dentists who have been granted privileges for a limited period of time by the chief medical staff officer on the recommendation of the chief of a particular department.

Tendinitis : Inflammation of tendons and their attachments.

Tendon : A band of tough white fibrous tissue that connects a muscle to a bone.

Tenesmus : Painful straining to empty the bowl or bladder, without success.

Tension Headache : A sensation of dull pain commonly associated with the stresses of everyday life but, when persistent, may be a presenting feature of an anxiety state or a depressive illness.

Tentative Diagnosis : See *Provisional Diagnosis*.

Terminal : An input-output unit by which a user communicates with a data processing system.

Terminal Decision : A decision that makes a final disposition of the choice of a best act.

Terminal Digit Filing : A method of medical record filing by the last digits of a number instead of by the first digits. The entire number is broken down into groups of twos or threes, with the last group being filed first.

Terminal Illness : An illness that finally leads to a patient's death after a more or less set period of time.

Term Neonate : Any neonate whose birth occurs from the beginning of the first day (267th day) of the 39th week, through the end of the last day of the 42nd week (294th day), following onset of the last menstrual period.

Terms of Trade : The ratio of a country's index of average export prices to its index of average import prices.

Tertiary Education : Education at the third level, such as universities, teachers colleges and higher professional schools — requiring as a minimum condition of admission the successful completion of education at the secondary level.

Tertiary Health Care : Specialized health care that requires highly specific facilities and the attention of highly specialized health workers (*e.g.* for neurosurgery or heart surgery).

Test : A process by which data are accumulated to serve as a basis for assessing the degree that an item or system meets, exceeds or fails to meet the technical or operational properties required of the system.

Testing Threshold : In diagnostic testing, the point at which the optimal decision is to perform a diagnostic test.

Test of Independence : A test for the independence of two variables on the basis of sample data.

Testosterone : The androgenic hormone formed in the testes which controls the development and maintenance of the male gonads and secondary sex characteristics.

Test-Retest (Reliability) : A measure of the degree to which an instrument or test provides a consistent measure of a characteristic on different (repeated) occasions.

Test Statistic : The specific statistic used to test the null hypothesis (*e.g.* the *t* statistic or chi-square statistic).

Test Tube Babies : Popular term for offspring of artificial insemination.

Tetanus : An infectious disease of the central nervous system caused by *Clostridium tetani,* and characterized by paroxysms of muscle spasm superimposed on an increased muscular rigidity.

Tetany : A disease characterized by intermittent fibrillary twitchings and spasm of muscles, usually caused by a fall in the ionic calcium concentration of the blood which may result from vitamin D deficiency.

Tetrachoric Correlation Coefficient : A measure of the strength of the relationship between two dichotomous variables, used when the distribution underlying both variables is assumed to be normal.

Tetralogy of Fallot : Congenital malformation of the heart, exhibiting four distinct defects.

Thalassaemia : A haemolytic anaemia found typically in peoples of Mediterranean origin due to a dominant Mendelian inherited abnormality of haemoglobin.

Thalidomide : A sedative that was withdrawn from use because of the high incidence of deformed foetuses it produced when given to pregnant women.

Thelarche : The beginning of breast development at puberty.

Thenar : Pertaining to the palm of the hand.

Theoretical Sampling Distribution : An estimate of an experimental sampling distribution that is determined mathematically (rather than by drawing repeated samples).

Therapy : Treatment of disease. Anything that is "therapeutic" is designed to help or heal.

Thermometer : An instrument for measuring temperature.

Thermostat : An apparatus for the automatic controlling of temperature.

Theta : In power analysis, an alternative hypothesis for the difference between two means that is *not* equal to zero and is expressed in raw units.

Third Party Payment : That type of payment utilized by those who spend a regular part of their income or work benefits on health care insurance and, in turn, receive full or partial payment for their health care.

Third Quartile : The 75th percentile.

Thoracocentesis : Puncture of the chest wall with a hallow needle for withdrawal of fluids.

Thoracoplasty : The surgical procedure of removing a varying number of ribs in order to induce collapse of the underlying lung.

Thoracoscope : An endoscope for examining the pleural cavity.

Thoracotomy : Surgical incision of the thoracic wall.

Threadworm : See *Pinworm*.

Threshold Model : A model for deciding when a diagnostic test should be ordered, as opposed to doing nothing or treating the patient without performing the test.

Thrombocytes : Blood *platelets* which help to initiate blood clotting.

Thrombocytopenia : A reduction in the number of platelets in the blood.

Thrombophlebitis : Inflammation of a vein combined with thrombus formation.

Thrombosis : The formation of a thrombus (a clot) in the circulation from the constituents of the blood.

Thrombus : A clot which forms in a blood vessel and remains at the site of attachment.

Thrush : Infection of the mucosa of the mouth and pharynx with *Candida albicans.*

Thyroidectomy : Surgical excision of the thyroid gland.

Thyroiditis : Acute or chronic inflammation of the thyroid gland.

Thyrotoxicosis (Hyperthyroidism) : The toxic condition induced by overaction of the thyroid gland, and characterized by nervousness, palpitations, loss of weight, excessive sweating and exophthalmos.

Thyroxine : The hormone released from the thyroid gland.

Tic : A repetitive twitching. **Tic douloureux,** trigeminal neuralgia.

Tick : A blood-sucking arthropod; some varieties are responsible for the transmission of disease to man and lower orders of animals.

Time, Access : The time interval between the instant at which data are called for from a storage device and the instant at which delivery is completed.

Time Cost : The cost individuals incur in being inactive through illness or in travelling to and waiting for health services.

Time Series : Any sequence of measurements taken on a variable process over time. Usually illustrated as a graph whose vertical coordinate gives a value of the random response plotted against time on the horizontal axis.

Time Sharing Operation : A system in which a number of users buy time and share the resources of a central computer.

Tincture : An alcoholic liquid containing the active principle of a vegetable drug in comparatively low concentration.

Tinea : Ringworm. A fungal infection of the skin or its appendages.

Tinnitus : Subjective sensation of noise in the ear.

Tipped Uterus : Forward, backward, or other displacement of the uterus form its theoretically ideal position.

Tissue : A conglomeration of similar cells and their intercellular substance.

Tissue Committee : Committee responsible for the review of surgical procedures in the facility.

Tissue Culture : A method of growing cells in a suitable nutrient in flasks or test tubes outside of the body, and of propagating viruses in the cells.

Titre : The amount of one substance which is equivalent to a stated amount of another. **Agglutination Titre,** the highest dilution of a serum that will produce clumping of the relevant micro-organisms.

Tolerance : A decrease in response to a drug dose that occurs with continued use. Increased doses of drugs are required to achieve the effects originally produced by lower doses.

Tolerance Limits : In matching, the range of values for a part of an identification code within which variation is disregarded—for example, treating all ages in any five-year age interval as the same.

Tomography : Sectional or body-section radiography. A technique whereby the shadow of a given plane can be clarified by a relative displacement of all other planes which are consequently blurred.

Tone : The basic tension of resting muscle. The quality of a sound Tonus.

Tonometer : An instrument for measuring internal pressures of the eyeball, used in the screening for glaucoma.

Tonsillitis : Inflammation of a tonsil, particularly the palatine tonsil.

Tonus : The slight degree of continuing tension present in muscle, and which is manifest in the resistance to stretching shown by healthy muscle.

Tophi : Masses of urate deposits in the external ear, joints, and other structures composed largely of cartilage; characteristic of gout.

Topography : The description of an anatomic region or a special part.

Torpor : A state of bodily and mental inactivity.

Torticollis : Wryneck. Spasmodic contraction of the muscles of the neck resulting in drawing of the head to one side.

Total Abortion Rate : The number of legal abortions performed on 1,000 females given their survival up to the age of 50, calculated from the age-specific abortion rates of the year of abortion.

Total Error : The difference between the estimate from a particular sample and the true value of the same characteristic. In other words, the sum of all the sources of error affecting such an estimate.

Total Fertility Rate : Average number of births to women living through child bearing ages under constant age-specific birth rates.

Total Inpatient Service Days : The sum of all inpatient/resident service days for each of the days in the period under consideration.

Total Length of Stay : The sum of the days' stay of any group of inpatients/residents discharged during a special period of time.

Total Per cent : In a cross-tabulation, the result of dividing a cell frequency by the total number of cases in the sample. Total per cents sum to 100% for the entire cross-tabulation.

Total Sum of Squares : The sum of the squared deviations of every raw score from the total mean of the study.

Total System Cost : The total research and development, and operating resource requirements (for a specified number of years) required to develop, procure, and operate, the particular system.

Touch Panel : A computer input device in which switches are activated by touching a sensitized surface.

Tourniquet : An instrument for the temporary arrest of haemorrhage by pressure on the bleeding blood vessel.

Toxaemia : The condition evoked by the presence of bacterial toxins in the circulating blood.

Toxic : Pertaining to a toxin (a poisonous substance). **Toxicity** refers to the state of being toxic or poisonous. **Toxicology** is the study of poisons.

Toxoid : A preparation containing detoxified toxin; employed to induce specific active resistance to the toxin, *e.g.* of diphtheria or tetanus bacilli.

Toxoplasmosis : The disease induced in man by infestation with *Toxoplasma gondii;* the congenital form may cause hydrocephaly in the foetus.

Tracer Conditions : Easily diagnosed, reasonably frequent illnesses whose outcomes are believed to be affected by health care and which, taken in aggregate, should reflect the gamut of patients and health problems encountered in a medical practical; used as an indicator to assess the quality of health care.

Tracheostomy : The surgical procedure of making an opening into the trachea for the insertion of a tube to maintain respiration.

Trachoma : A contagious disease of the eyes, caused by viruses which attack the lining membranes of the lids and eyes.

Traction : The act of drawing or pulling (as in the case of a long bone by means of pins).

Traditional Fuels : Includes fuelwood, charcoal, bagasse, and animal and vegetable wastes.

Traffic Accidents : Accidents on streets, roads, and highways involving drivers, passengers, pedestrians or vehicles (passenger cars, buses, trucks, etc.).

Tranquillizer : A calming agent : A general term for several classes of drugs used to relieve anxiety (minor tranquillizers) or to diminish psychotic symptoms (major tranquillizers).

Transaction : A short interaction between a computer and an operator for a specific purpose, such as recording a payment or entering a name.

Transcribe : To transfer data from one data machine to another, converting them as necessary for acceptance by the receiving medium.

Transducer : A device which converts energy from one form to another, *e.g.* a quartz crystal embedded in mercury can change electrical energy to sound energy as is done in some delay lines in computer storage systems.

Transfer : Movement of a patient from one treatment service or location to another.

Transfer Data : An abstract or summary of an individual patient care plan to accompany the patient to another care facility.

Transformation : The act of replacing a data set with the equivalent values in another measurement system (for example, replacing the original values with their logarithms which will make a skewed data set normal).

Transformed Score : A score that has been altered mathematically to show its standing relative to a specified group.

Transfusion : The introduction of fluid directly into the circulation. This may be blood, blood substitutes, normal saline, or other solutions.

Transmission of Infectious Agents : Any mechanism by which an infectious agent is spread from a source or reservoir to a person. These mechanisms are : direct transmission, indirect transmission, and transmission by airborne droplets and dust.

Transplantation : The process of transferring tissue from one site to another or organs or tissue from one individual to another.

Transport Accident : Any accident involving a device designed primarily for, or being used at the time primarily for, conveying persons or goods from one place to another.

Transposition : Change of position. Displacement of an organ to the opposite side.

Transsexual : A person affected by *transsexualism*—a disturbance of gender identity in which the person wishes to be of the opposite sex, often seeking hormonal and surgical treatment to achieve this goal.

Transudate : A morbid accumulation of fluid due to a hydrostatic imbalance between the intravascular and extravascular components of the body.

Transvestite : A person who derives sexual pleasure from dressing in the clothes of the opposite sex.

Trauma : Injury, wound.

Traumatic Procedures : Procedures that are invasive, including non-surgical procedures that utilize cutdowns, that cause tissue damage (*e.g.* irradiation), or introduce some toxic or noxious substance (*e.g.* caustic test reagents).

Treatment : The means employed in the management and care of patients.

Treatment Effect : The presence of differences in mean performance between treatment groups resulting from genuine differences in treatment effectiveness.

Treatment Threshold : In diagnostic testing, the point at which the optimal decision is to treat the patient without first performing a diagnostic test.

Treatment Variance : In ANOVA, the amount of variance among the sample means due to the independent variable.

Trematoda : The class of the phylum platyhelminthes. Also known as *flukes*.

Tremor : Involuntary rhythmic quivering or trembling.

Trench Mouth : (Vincent's infection). Painful, swollen, foul-smelling inflammation of the mouth and gums.

Trend : The smooth upward or downward movement of a time series over a long period of time.

Trend Line : The line that best fits the distribution of a set of values plotted on two axes.

Trepanning : Cutting a button of bone out of the skull with a *trephine*.

Trepanoma : A tribe of spiral microbes responsible for a number of infectious diseases, including syphilis.

Trephine : A surgical instrument to removing a circular disc—usually of bone from the skull.

Trial : An experiment involving humans, commonly called a clinical trial. It is also a replication (repetition) of an experiment.

Trichinosis, Trichiniasis : The disease caused by *Trichinella spiralis*, characterized by muscular pains, eosinophilia and fever.

Trichobezoar : A ball of hair formed into a mass in the stomach.

Trichomoniasis : Infestation with *Trichomonas vaginalis*, usually manifested by vaginitis in women and urethritis in men.

Trichophytosis : Ringworm of the scalp.

Trigger Finger : A condition in which efforts to unbend a finger are at first unsuccessful, but it is soon straightened with a snap or a jerk, like the release of a trigger.

Trimester : Three months, or one-third of the nine months of pregnancy.

Triplet : One of three individuals produced at the same birth.

Trismus : Lockjaw. Inability to open the mouth, as in tetanus.

Trocar : A perforating instrument for puncturing a cavity to release fluid.

Tropical Ulcer : Chronic, tissue-destroying ulcer of the lower leg or foot, caused by a spirochaete.

True Negative : A test result that is negative in a person who does not have the disease.

True Positive : A test result that is positive in a patient who has the disease.

True Treatment Effect : The difference in the mean performance of two treatments that would be observed if the treatments could be administered to every individual in the population under study, expressed in standardized units.

Truncated Range : When one end of a distribution of sample scores is arbitrarily cut off. In a correlational analysis, if one variable has a truncated range, the correlation of the sample will tend to underestimate the population correlation.

Truss : An instrument for supporting a hernia and preventing the egress of organs in the affected cavity.

Trypanosomiasis : African sleeping sickness, produced by the bite of an infected insect.

T Score : A converted standard score such that the mean equals 50 and the standard deviation equals 10. T scores, thus, range from a low of 20 to a high of 80.

***t*-Test :** The statistical test for comparing a mean with a norm or for comparing two means with small sample size (less than 30); also used for testing whether a correlation coefficient or a regression coefficient is zero.

Tubal Ligation (Salpingectomy) : An operation for sterilization of women, by cutting and tying the oviducts.

Tubal Pregnancy : Implantation of a fertilized egg in the walls of the Fallopian tube instead of in the uterus.

Tubercle : A small nodule or prominence.

Tuberculin : The name originally given by Koch to a preparation derived from *Mycobacterium tuberculosis,* and intended for the treatment and diagnosis of tuberculosis.

Tuberculosis : The disease caused by infection with *Mycobacterium tuberculosis* (Commonly called T.B.).

Tukey's HSD (Honestly Significant Difference) : A multiple comparison technique developed by J.W. Tukey for establishing whether or not the differences among various sample means are significant. The test is performed *after* the ANOVA when the *F* ratio is significant.

Tularaemia : An infectious disease of rodents due to *Pasteurella tularensis,* transmitted to man by ticks, and presenting a clinical picture comparable to that of plague.

Tumefaction : Swelling.

Tumour : A new growth of tissue in which cell multiplication is uncontrolled and progressive. See also *Neoplasm.*

Tunnel Vision : A restriction of peripheral vision, occurring in retinitis pigmentosa and advanced chronic glaucoma.

Turner's Syndrome : A congenital condition in which the ovaries do not mature or produce egg cells.

Turnover Interval : The mean number of days a bed is not occupied between the admissions.

Turnover Rate : The number of separations (discharges, deaths and transfers) divided by the mean number of available beds.

Tussis : A cough.

Twilight State : A state of impaired consciouness in which complex, irrational behaviour may occur of which no memory is subsequently retained; associated with epilepsy, alcohol intoxication, and delirious conditions.

Twin : One of two offspring born as the result of one pregnancy.

Two-Point Scale : If each case is classified into one of two categories (*e.g.* yes/no, male/female, dead/alive), the variable is a two-point scale. For analytic purposes, two-point scales can be treated as nominal, ordinal or interval scales.

Two-Sample *t* Test : The statistical test used to test the null hypothesis that two independent (or unrelated) groups have the same mean.

Two-tailed Test : A directional test in which the alternative hypothesis specifies a deviation from the null hypothesis in either direction. The critical region is located in both ends (or tails) of the sampling distribution.

Two-way Analysis of Variance : ANOVA with two independent variables. A statistical method requiring independent samples that is used to determine whether population means are related to two factors.

Tympanitis : Taut distension of the abdomen by intestinal gases or fluids, bloating.

Tympanoplasty : Surgical reconstruction of the middle ear.

Type I Error : The error that results if a true null hypothesis is rejected, or if a difference is concluded when there is no difference.

Type II Error : The error that results if a false null hypothesis is not rejected, or if a difference is not detected when there is a difference.

Type A Behaviour : A lifestyle said to be associated with an increased risk of coronary heart disease; characterized by intense, sustained energy and drive, a high level of competitive spirit, and hostility when frustrated over objectives or deadlines.

Type of Care : The facilities and personnel available for health care, and more importantly, the objective of the care.

Typhoid Fever : An acute infectious fever due to *Salmonella typhi,* and characterized by continued fever, splenomegaly and rose spots.

Typhus : One of a group of related infections caused by *Rickettsiae,* and characterized by fever, skin rash, etc.

U

Ulcer : An excavation of the surface of an organ or tissue, produced by sloughing of necrotic inflammatory tissue.

Ulcerative Colitis : Inflammation of the colon and rectum, characterized by sores or ulcers inside the tube, and bloody diarrhea.

Ultramicroscopic : Too small to be seen with the ordinary light microscope.

Ultrasonography : The visualization of the deep structures of the body by recording the reflection of ultrasonic waves directed into the tissue.

Umbilical Cord : The long flexible tube which is attached to the placenta at one end and to the abdomen of the foetus at another.

Umbilical Hernia : A protrusion of the intestines through a weakness in the abdominal wall in the region of the navel, not uncommon in infants.

Umbilicated : Depressed like a navel.

Umbilicus : The navel; the scar marking the site of attachment of the umbilical cord in the foetus.

Unbiased Statistic : A term used to describe a statistic whose mean, based on a large number of samples, is equal to the population parameter, it estimates, *i.e.* E (estimator) = parameter.

Uncinaria : Hookworms.

Uncontrolled Study : An experimental study that has no control subjects.

Under-5 Mortality Rate : An indicator of the status of perinatal conditions to which mothers are subjected and the effects of environmental factors in early childhood. It is calculated by dividing the number of under-5 deaths in the given year by the total number of under-5 children at the middle of the year; expressed per 1,000 per year.

Under-5 Proportionate Mortality : An indicator of the status of perinatal conditions and the effects of environmental factors in early childhood. The proportion is calculated by dividing the under-5 deaths during a given period by the total number of deaths during the same period.

Underlying Cause of Death : The disease or injury which initiated the train of morbid events leading directly to death, or the circumstances of the accident or violence which produced the fatal injury.

Underreporting : Failure to identify and/or count all cases, leading to reduction of numerator in a rate.

Underweight : The percentage of children under age five who are below minus two standard deviations from the median birth weight for age of the reference population.

Undescended Testicles : See *Cryptorchidism.*

Undine : A small glass flask use for irrigating the eye.

Undulant Fever : See *Brucellosis.*

Unemployment : All persons above a specified age who are not in paid employment or self-employed, but are available and have taken specific steps to seek paid employment or self-employment.

Ungual : Pertaining to the nails.

Unguentum : An ointment.

Unilateral : Affecting only one side.

Unimodal Distribution : A distribution of scores in which only one mode (most frequently occurring score) is present. When graphed as a frequency polygon it appears as a pronounced peak.

Unintentional Injury : Injury that is not inflicted by deliberate means.

Uniovular : Pertaining to, or originating from a single egg, an identical twin.

Unique Factor : The factor which is believed to affect only a single observed variable; often stands for all the independent factors that are unique to a variable.

Unit : The term applied to a quantity recognized as a standard for measurement. A single item. S.I. Units : *Systéme International d'Unités,* any of the metric units in replacement of the CGS unit system.

Unit, Arithmetic : The unit of a computing system that contains the circuits that perform arithmetic operations.

Unit Control : The unit of a computing system that contains the circuits that interpret and control the execution of instructions.

Unit Cost : The total cost of an activity divided by the number of units of output produced. Also known as *average cost.*

Unit-Normal Linear Loss Integral : A table of values that facilitates calculation of certain EMVs (Expected Monetary Values) for continuous function decision problems.

Unit Numbering : A system in which only one number is assigned to the patient's record and is retained permanently.

Unit Record System : A method that compiles all information on a single patient or subject and records it in one document and file folder.

Units of Observation : The types of elements being studied or observed. Individuals are most often the unit of observation, but sometimes collections or aggregates—such as families, census tracts, or states—are the unit of observation.

Univariate Approach : A procedure for repeated-measures analysis of variance that is based on sums of squares and requires more variance-covariance assumptions than the multivariate or adjusted univariate approaches to repeated-measures analysis of variance.

Univariate Distribution : A frequency distribution based on one variable.

Universe : The total number of items under discussion, from which a sample is drawn.

UNIX : An operating system developed by Bell Labs for mini- and micro-computers which includes many useful features, particularly multiprogramming and multiusers.

Unverified Suicides : Deaths regarding which there is doubt as to whether the outcome was intentional or not.

Update : Put into a master file changes required by current information or transactions.

Upper Real Limit : The upper end point of a class interval in a grouped frequency distribution.

Upper Respiratory Tract Infection (URTI, URI) : Infection of nasal passages or throat above the lungs.

Upper Tail Probability : A probability calculated by computing an area in the upper tail (the right tail) of a distribution.

Uraemia : The retention of excessive by-products of protein metabolism (urea, etc.) in the blood and the toxic condition produced thereby, because of kidney failure.

Urbanization : The growth in the size of cities, the number of cities, and the proportion of the population living in urban locations.

Urban Population : Percentage of the population living in urban areas as defined according to the national definition used in the most recent population census.

Urethritis : Inflammation of the urethra (the passage through which urine is discharged from the bladder to the exterior of the body).

Uricaemia : Excessive amounts of uric acid in the blood.

Urinalysis : Laboratory analysis of a urine specimen.

Urodynia : Pain on urination.

Urogenital : Pertaining to the urinary and genital apparatus.

Urogram : X-ray visualization of the urinary tract made by injecting a radiopaque substance.

Urolithiasis : The formation of urinary calculi, or the condition associated with urinary calculi (stones).

Urology : The branch of medicine dealing with the urinary system in the female and genitourinary tract in the male. Urologist : a specialist in urology.

Uroscopy : Examination of urine.

Urticaria : Hives, a vascular reaction of the skin marked by transient appearance of red and slightly elevated patches, and often attended by severe itching.

Uterine Displacement : See *Tipped Uterus*.

Utility : (1) A personal subjective value of a tangible or intangible commodity. (2) The value of different outcomes in a decision tree.

Utility Function : A function that incorporates attitude toward risk in decision-making under uncertainty.

Utilization : The promotion of national and local acceptance of a technology, its proper application, production, and distribution to the users of instruments or other material when needed, and the monitoring of its effectiveness.

Utilization Review : Review to assure that a hospital's level of care is medically necessary, meets professionally recognized standards of care, and is delivered in the most cost-effective manner.

Utilization Review Committee : Committee which reviews all aspects of care in order to assure high-quality care through the effective use of equipment, personnel, materials and the facility as a whole.

Utopia : Any idea or proposal that may be desirable but is impractical or unrealizable; any visionary scheme for a perfect society.

***U*-Value** : The test statistic used in the Mann-Whitney *U* test.

Uveitis : Non-pus forming inflammation of the uvea, the iris and associated eye structures.

V

Vaccination : Procedures for immunization against infectious disease.

Vaccine : A preparation containing whole micro-organisms (killed or living) or a fraction of the organisms possessing immunizing antigen; employed to induce specific active immunity.

Vaccinia : Pox virus used as live virus vaccine against smallpox (commonly thought to have originated from cowpox as described by Jenner).

Vaginismus : Painful spasm of the vagina on attempted coitus.

Vaginitis : Inflammation of the vagina, characterized by discharge and discomfort.

Vagotomy : Surgical division of the vagus nerve.

Validation : The process of establishing that a method is sound.

Valid Criteria : Standards stated in measurable rather than descriptive terms, precise enough to permit accurate evaluation. Statements of optimal achievable care. Measures of quality.

Validity : The property of a measurement that measures the characteristic it purports to measure.

Value : The assessment of the contribution (to the accomplishment of the objective) of the generally non-quantifiable characteristics of an alternative.

Valvotomy : Surgical operation for widening a stenosed valve.

Vaporizer : An instrument for producing a fine, vaporized spray for inhalation. An atomizer.

Variability : The extent to which the scores in a specified group differ from one another, or how spread out or scattered the scores are. Also known as *dispersion* or *spread.*

Variability Measures : Measures that give information regarding individual differences, or how persons or events vary in their measured scores. The three most important measures of variability are the *range,* the *standard deviation,* and the *variance* (the standard deviation squared).

Variable : Anything that varies and can be measured, *i.e.* any characteristics that may fluctuate from one individual to another. Hypotheses usually contain an independent variable (cause) and a dependent variable (effect).

Variable Data : The phrase used in quality control to refer to measured data, that is, data from some continuous random variable.

Variance : A measure of the variability of the scores in a specified group, or how much the scores differ from one another; the square of the standard deviation.

Variance-Covariance Assumptions : Assumptions about covariances of random variables that are required for repeated-measures analysis of variance.

Variation Analysis : Identification of conformance to and variations from the audit (or valid) criteria. It requires explicit justification for all variations that are clinically acceptable, identification of problems in the provision of patient care, and attribution of the problems to their source.

Variation Justification : An acceptable reason why a given finding or element is not in agreement with the norm or standard.

Varicella : Chickenpox

Varices : Varicose veins.

Varicocele : Varicosity of the testicular veins accompanied with scrotal swelling.

Varicose Vein : Unnatural and permanently dilated or distended vein. **Varicotomy** : excision of a varicose vein.

Varimax : A method of orthogonal rotation which simplifies the factor structure by maximizing the variance of a column of the pattern matrix.

Variola : Smallpox.

Vascular : Pertaining to or abundant in vessels, especially blood vessels.

Vasectomy : Surgical excision of the whole, or part, of the vas deferens (the semen-carrying duct of the testis).

Vasoconstrictor : A drug or natural body substance or mechanism that constricts small blood vessels.

Vasodilator : An agent that dilates small blood vessels so that more blood flows through them.

Vasomotor : Pertaining to mechanisms that controls dilation or constriction of walls of blood vessels.

VDRL Test : A screening test for syphilis using blood serum (*V*enereal *D*isease *R*esearch *L*aboratory).

Vector : (1) The "vehicle" by which an infectious agent is transferred from an infected to a susceptible host. (2) A quantity that has both magnitude and direction.

Vegan : An extreme vegetarian who does not even take milk, butter, cheese or eggs.

Venereal : Relating to, or propagated by, sexual intercourse. Venereologist : a practitioner who specializes in venereal disease.

Venesection : Bloodletting; same as **Phlebotomy**.

Venipuncture : Surgical puncture of a vein.

Venn Diagram : A diagram portraying graphically the extent to which two or more quantities or concepts are mutually inclusive and mutually exclusive.

Venoclysis : Injection of fluids by vein.

Venography : Visualization of the veins by radiography, with or without the injection of radio-opaque substances.

Venom : Poison, particularly that secreted by snakes and the like.

Ventilation : The process of change of air. The exchange of air in the lungs.

Ventouse : Vacuum extractor; used in obstetrics as a means of facilitating the birth of the child.

Ventral : The belly side; the aspect of a part directed toward the belly.

Ventriculogram : An X-ray of the brain taken after introducing air or a contrast medium into certain ventricles.

Vermicide : An antihelminth. An agent or drug that kills worms.

Vermiform : Worm-shaped.

Vernix Caseosa : A greasy, cheesy substance that covers the skin of the foetus, removed at the first cleansing.

Verruca : A wart.

Version : Turning, manipulation of the foetus in the uterus to attain a better position for delivery.

Vertebra : (pl. vertebrae). One of the 33 bones which constitute the backbone.

Vertex : The highest point of the skull, the topmost part of the head.

Vertigo : A sensation of rotation or movement of one's self or of one's surroundings in any plane.

Vesicant : An agent that induces blistering.

Vesicle : A small sac containing fluid, a tiny bladder, like a skin blister.

Viability : Ability to remain alive in the free state.

Viable : Able to maintain an independent existence; able to live after birth.

Vial : A small bottle. Phial.

Vibrissae : Hairs in the nose. Also, a cat's whiskers.

Victim : Person who is the target of violence or abuse.

Victimology : The study of the victim of maltreatment including the immediate reaction to the traumatic event and various other post-traumatic issues.

Villi : Minute fingerlike projections from the surface of a mucous membrane.

Vincent's Infection : See *Trench Mouth*.

Vineland Scale : An age scale, similar in design to the Stanford-Binet test, that covers the entire period from birth to adulthood and purports to measure socio-emotional development in terms of Social Quotient.

Violence : The intentional use of, or threat of use of, physical force against another person or against oneself, which results in or has a high likehood of resulting in injury or death.

Virgin : A woman who has never had sexual intercourse.

Virgin Population : A population that has never been exposed to a particular infectious agent.

Virilism : Masculinity. The development of masculine traits in the female.

Virology : The study of viruses and virus diseases.

Virulence : The degree of pathogenicity of an infectious agent, indicated by case fatality rates and/or its ability to invade and damage tissues of the host.

Viruses : Molecules that cause disease.

Visceroptosis : Sagging of abdominal organs from their normal position.

Viscid : Sticky, adhesive.

Visiting Hours : Designated hours during the day when patients in a hospital are allowed to receive visitors; often extend from 11.00 A.M. to 12.30 P.M. and from 4.00 P.M. to 7.00 P.M.

Visual Field : The area of physical space seen when the gaze is fixed straight ahead.

Visual Purple : A pigment produced by rods of the retina, essential for good vision in dim light.

Vital Depression : A characteristic morbid change in vital feeling that is near physical, often sharply localized, melancholy, allied with other bodily distress.

Vital Events : Significant major events within the lifetime of individuals. These include live births, deaths, foetal deaths, marriages, divorces, adoptions, legitimations, recognitions, annulments and legal separations.

Vital Events Registration : Legal registration, statistical recording and reporting of the occurrence of, and the collection, compilation, presentation, analysis and distribution of statistics pertaining to vital events.

Vital Records : Certificates of birth, death, marriage, and divorce required for legal and demographic purposes.

Vital Signs : The indications of life in a patient. The blood pressure, the pulse or heartbeat, and the temperature are major vital signs that are checked regularly.

Vital Statistics : Systematically tabulated information concerning births, marriages, divorces, separations, and deaths based on registrations of these vital events.

Vitamin : An organic substance present in minute amounts in natural foodstuffs, which is essential for normal nutrition.

Vitiligo : Leucoderma. A condition characterized by white patches of skin.

Vitreous Humour : Transparent, colourless, soft gelatinous material which fills the eyeball behind the lens.

Voluntary Hospital : A private, non-profit hospital that is financed by private contributions and sometimes by government grants.

Volvulus : A twisting of the bowel on itself, resulting in obstruction.

Vomiting : The forceful expulsion of the contents of the stomach through the mouth.

Voyeurism : A disorder of sexual preference consisting of a recurrent or persistent tendency to look at people engaging in sexual or intimate behaviour such as undressing.

Vulvovaginitis : Inflammation of the vulva and vagina.

W

Waiting Time : The time until the occurrence of some event.

Waiver : The voluntary relinquishing of a known right.

Wall Eye : Outward turning of an eye; divergent squint, a condition of ocular muscle imbalance.

Ward : A large room in a hospital, with beds for the accommodation of many patients. **Isolation Ward :** One for isolation of persons having or suspected of having infectious disease.

Wart : An epidermal tumour of viral origin. Verruca.

Wash : A solution used for cleansing or bathing a part, as an eye or the mouth.

Washout Phase : In a clinical or drug trial, that stage or phase when treatment is withdrawn so that its effects disappear and the patient's characteristics return to their baseline state.

Wassermann Test : A complement fixation test for the diagnosis of syphilis by determining the presence of syphilitic antibodies in the blood serum.

Waste Recycling : The reuse of material that diverts it from the waste stream, except for recycling within industrial plants and the reuse of material as fuel. The recycling rate is the ratio of the quantity recycled to the apparent consumption.

Water Bag : The fluid filled amnion surrounding the foetus in human beings and other placental mammals.

Water-borne Diseases : Diseases spread or transmitted by drinking water such as cholera, typhoid, and hepatitis.

Water Resources : The average annual flow of rivers and aquifers generated from endogenous precipitation.

WBC. : *W*hite *B*lood *C*ell; white blood (cell) count.

Weal : A well-defined, slightly raised, flat lesion with reddened margins, caused by the release of histamine. A manifestation of the sting of an insect.

Wean : To discontinue breast and substitute other feeding habits.

Webbed Fingers : Connection of adjacent fingers (or toes) by a thin fold of skin between them.

Weighted Average : A number formed by multiplying each number in a set of numbers by a value called a weight, adding the resulting products, and then dividing by the sum of the weights.

Weighted Data : Forces (multipliers, constants) applied to data when one wishes to adjust the impact of cases (*e.g.* persons) in the analysis, *e.g.* to take account of the number of population units that each case represents.

Weighted Mean : The mean of two or more individual means in which the individual means are weighted according to their respective sample sizes.

Weil Disease : An acute feverish illness caused by spirochaetes; also called *infectious jaundice*. A severe form of Leptospirosis.

Welch's *t* Test : The separate-variance *t* test.

Welfare Expenditure : Expenditures on assistance delivered to persons or groups with special needs, such as the young, the old, or the handicapped.

Well Newborn : Newborn delivered at term, under sterile conditions, with no diseases, conditions, disorders, syndromes, injuries, malformations or defects diagnosed, and no operations (other than routine circumcision, according to tradition) performed.

Wen : A sebaceous or epidermal inclusion cyst.

Wet-Nurse : A women who suckles infants other than her own.

Wetzel Grid : A chart for plotting, comparing, and projecting the height, weight, and other growth aspects of children.

Wheals : Hives, temporary skin swellings resembling mosquito bites, but often much larger.

Wheeze : To breathe noisily and with difficulty. The sound produced by obstructed breathing, usually of a whistling character.

Whiplash : An injury to the spine and spinal cord due to sudden extension of the neck.

Whipworms : Slender worms which inhabit the caecum of dogs, pigs, sheep and goats.

Whites : Vaginal discharge.

Whitlow : A malignant tumour of the nail bed characterized by formation of melanotic tissue.

WHO World Health Organization : An international agency based in Geneva, associated with the United Nations and devoting itself to promoting health and hygiene in all countries of the world.

WHO General Programme of Work : The programme constitutes WHO's support for national, regional, and global strategies and plans of action for the attainment of health for all by the year 2000. Each programme covers a period of six years.

W.H.R. : *W*aist-to-*h*ip *r*atio. The ratio of waist and hip measurement and a measure of abdominal obesity (a ratio of 0.89 for men and 0.76 for women means acceptable weight).

Whooping Cough : One of the commonest infectious diseases of childhood, due to infection of the respiratory tract with *Bordetella pertussis,* and characterized by a cough terminating in a typical whoop (crowing inspiration), pertussis.

Widal Test : An antibody test of blood for diagnosis of typhoid fever.

Wilcoxon *T* Test : A non-parametric test on ordinal data of the hypothesis of difference between two sample groups when the selections are correlated (as in the matched-subjects design). It is the ordinal counterpart of the paired *t* test.

Wilk's Lambda : A test statistic used in the multivariate approach to repeated measures analysis of variance.

Wilm's Tumour : A malignant tumour of the kidney occurring in children.

Withdrawal State : A group of symptoms (sweating, depression, malaise, instability, muscle aches and twitching) of variable degree of severity occurring on absolute or relative withdrawal of a substance after persistent use of that substance.

Within-Group Variation : The variation of scores within a group. Reflects variation that cannot be explained by the experimental treatment.

Within Subjects *F* Ratio : Statistical test of the hypothesis of difference between sample means, whose sample selection is not independent. It is used when samples are correlated, as in repeated-measure designs, and the data are in at least interval form.

Within-Treatment Variation : Variation of the individual observations within each treatment from their respective means X, $\overline{X}$, etc.

Womb : The uterus.

Word : In computer terminology, an ordered set of characters which occupies one storage location and is treated by the computer circuits as a unit and transferred as such. Word lengths may be fixed or variable depending on the particular computer.

Work Condition Indicators : Indicators reflecting the availability of work, the level of unemployment or underemployment, the percentage of women in the labour force and the prevalence of disability preventing gainful employment.

Work-related Injuries : Those recordable injuries resulting from accidents occurring at the place of work and resulting in death, personal injury or acute disease.

Workshop : A seminar or series of meetings for intensive study, work discussion, etc. in some field (*e.g.* a workshop on family planning methods).

Worm Count : A method of surveillance of helminth infection of the gut that depends upon counts of worms, or their cysts or ova, in quantitatively titrated samples of faeces.

Wound : A sudden breach in the tissues of the body produced by physical means.

Wrist Drop : Drooping of the hand at the wrist due to paralysis or injury of muscles or tendons which extend the fingers and hands.

Wrong-Way Match : A one-way match that yields a match rate and completeness estimate irrelevant to the question being studied.

Wryneck : See *Torticollis*.

X

Xanthelasma : Xanthoma affecting the eyelids, marked by soft yellowish spots or plaques, most commonly in elderly women.

Xanthoma : A small yellow-orange focal accumulation of fat-laden papules found in the skin.

Xanthomatosis : A condition attended by means of yellowish deposits in tissues due to some disturbance of cholesterol and lipid metabolism.

Xanthopsia : "Yellow vision", a condition in which objects look yellow. It sometimes accompanies jaundice.

Xanthosis : Yellow discoloration of the skin, due to eating excessive amounts of yellow vegetable.

***X* Chromosome :** One of the two sex determining chromosomes in the germ cells of most animals and a few plants (the other being *Y*); carried by the eggs or ova.

Xenobiotic : A foreign compound that is metabolized in the body; examples include many pesticides, some food additives and a number of other complex organic compounds.

Xenodiagnosis : Detection of a (human) pathogenic organism by allowing a non-infected vector (*e.g.* mosquito) to consume infected material, and then examining this vector for evidence of the pathogen.

Xenophobia : Morbid fear of meeting strangers or foreigners.

Xeroderma : A hereditary condition characterized by dryness of the skin. **Xeroderma pigmentosum**, a congenital condition in which there is an inborn susceptibility to sunlight.

Xerophthalmia : A dry, lustreless condition of the conjunctiva due either to local infection or lack of vitamin A. Xerosis.

Xerosis : Abnormal dryness, as of the eye or skin.

Xerostomia : Dryness of the mouth due to inadequate salivary secretion.

Xerox : A trademark for a process for copying graphic or printed material by xerography. To reproduce by xerography, to make a photostat copy.

Xiphoid : Shapped like a sword; applies to the structure at the lower tip of the breastbone.

X-Linked : Transmitted by genes on the *X* chromosome. Sex-linked.

X-rays : Electromagnetic radiations of short wave-length, characterized by their ability to penetrate opaque matter; widely used in medicine for study, diagnosis, and treatment of certain organic disorders, especially of internal structures of the body.

X-ray Therapy : Medical treatment by controlled use of X-rays.

Xylene : Dimethylbenzene. Used as a solvent and clarifier in microbiology. Xylol.

Xylulose : A pentose sugar excreted in the urine in pentosuria.

Xyster : A surgical instrument for scraping bones.

Y

Yardstick : Any test or standard used in measuring, judging, etc.

Yates' Correction : The (correcting) process of subtracting 0.5 from the numerator at each term in the chi-square value for 2×2 tables prior to squaring the term.

Yaws : A tropical infectious disease caused by a spirochete (*Treponema pertenue*) and characterized by typical skin eruptions followed by destructive lesions of the skin and bones.

***Y* Chromosome :** One of the two sex determining chromosomes in the germ cells of most animals and a few plants (the other being *X*) : carried by the spermatozoa.

Yeast : The name applied to various species of saccharomyces; rich source of some members of the vitamin B complex (*e.g.* thiamine, riboflavin, nicotinic acid); fermenters of carbohydrates and a few species pathogenic for man.

Yield : In epidemiology, the number or proportion of cases of a condition accurately identified by a screening test.

***Y* Intercept :** In regression, the point where the regression line crosses the *Y* axis. The *Y* intercept is the predicted value of *Y* for an *X* value of zero.

Yellow Fever : An acute, infectious tropical disease caused by a virus transmitted by the bite of the yellow-fever mosquito *(Aides aegypti)* and characterized by fever, jaundice and vomiting.

Yellow Spot : The macula lutea, the small spot near the center of the retina which is the focus of all finely detailed seeing.

Yoga : A system of exercising involving prescribed postures and controlled breathing, etc.

Yoghurt: A thick, semi-solid food made from milk fermented by a bacterium *(Lactobacillus bulgaricus)* believed to have a beneficial effect on the intestines.

Yolk : The protein and fat contents of the egg or ovum, serving as nourishment for the growing embryo.

YPLL : *Y*ears of *P*otential *L*ife *L*ost. See *Potential Years of Life Lost.*

Z

Z Distribution : The normal distribution where the mean is equal to zero and the standard deviation equal to 1.00. Also called the *Standard Normal Distribution.*

Zero Correlation : No relationship between the *X* and *Y* variables.

Zero-population Growth : Absence of any growth in the population.

Zero-Time Shift : A shift or movement backwards (*i.e.* towards the starting point of a disease), of time between onset and detection, that may accompany use of a disease screening procedure.

Zoning : In serology, the occurrence of a stronger fixation of complement in a lesser amount of suspected serum.

Zonules : Tiny sling-like processes which suspend the crystalline lens of the eye.

Zonulysis : A technique of dissolving the zonules with a specific enzyme to loosen the lens for extraction in selected cases of cataract surgery.

Zografting : The grafting of animal tissue.

Zooid : A comparatively independent animal organism produced by other than sexual methods, as by fission, germination, etc.

Zoolagnia : Sexual attraction towards animals.

Zoology: A branch of biology, that deals with animals, their life, structure, growth, classification, etc.

Zoonosis : An infection or infectious disease transmissable under natural conditions from vertebrate animals to man (*e.g.* rabies, plague), may be enzootic or epizootic.

Zoopsia : Seeing animals (*e.g.* snakes, insects), typically as part of delirium tremens or other substance-induced confusional or hallucinatory states.

Zooplankton : Minute animal organisms floating freely in practically all natural waters.

Zootoxin : A toxic substance of animal origin, *e.g.* venom of snakes, spiders, and scorpions.

Zoster : Shingles.

***Z*-Plasty** : Repair of skin defect by the transposition of two triangular folds, for relaxation of scar contracture.

Z* Ratio** : The test statistic used in the ***Z-test. It is formed by subtracting the hypothesized mean from the observed mean and dividing by the standard error of the mean.

***Z* Score (Standard Score)** : A transformed raw score that indicates the number of standard deviation units the raw score is from the mean of the distribution. The normal deviate *z*, has a mean equal to 0, and a standard deviation equal to 1.00.

***z* Test** : A significance test used to decide if a sample mean comes from a population with a specified norm (or mean), for comparing two means for large samples (over 30).

***Z* Transformation** : A transformation that changes a normally distributed variable with mean *X* and standard deviation *s* to the *z* distribution with mean zero and standard deviation 1.00.

Zygote : A cell formed by the union of male and female gametes; fertilized egg cell before cleavage.

Zygoma : The cheekbone.

Zymogen : An inactive antecedent form of an active enzyme that becomes functional by the action of an appropriate kinase or other activator.

Zymolysis : Fermentation of digestion by means of an enzyme.

Zymosis : A process, like fermentation, by which infectious diseases (*e.g.* smallpox) were formerly believed to be developed.

APPENDICES

APPENDIX-I

LIST OF SYMBOLS

Symbol	Meaning
$=$	is approximately equal to
$\geq$	is greater than or equal to, *i.e.*, 4>3
$\leq$	is less than or equal to, *i.e.*, 3<4
$>>$	is much greater than
$\pm$	plus or minus, usually followed by standard error
$\neq$	is not equal to
$\simeq$	approximately equal to
Σ	the sum of
∂	symbol indicating "derivative of...with respect to..."
[ ]	sum of terms inside the brackets, expressed as deviations from their arithmetic means
$\lvert\ \rvert$	absolute value of the terms enclosed between vertical lines
!	factorial; $n! = n\,(n-1)\ldots.!$
$-$	bar over a symbol, denoting its mean, *i.e* $\overline{X}$
^	hat; used to indicate an estimate of the term it covers, *i.e.* $\hat{p}$ (a sample proportion)
∞	infinity
α	error of the first kind (Type I error)
b_1	the sample regression slope
β	error of the second type (Type II error)
β_1	the population regression slope
χ^2	Chi-square statistic in a test of independence of goodness of fit
η	an inverse function of the variance in a regression with a zero intercept

θ	factor in a censored sample
λ	ratio of the standard deviation about a linear regression to its slope
μ	population mean
π	the geometric constant 3.14159
n	the number of observations
P	probability or level of significance
Q_r	a fixed set of weights in an index number formula
Q_n	quantity in a non-base period in an index number formula
Q_o	quantity in a base period in an index number formula
r	correlation coefficient between two variables
r_r	rank correlation coefficient
ρ	population correlation coefficient
ρ^2	population coefficient of determination
S	sample space
SI	seasonal index
σ	standard deviation of a population
σ^2	the population variance
$\sigma_{\bar{x}}$	standard error of the mean
t	the t-statistic, according to the Student's t distribution
$\hat{\theta}$	estimator of θ
T	overall total
T	Wilcoxon test statistic for comparing two samples
u	grouping unit in a coded variate
V	variance
W	weight applied to an observation
$\bar{\bar{X}}$	grand (arithmetic) mean of all observations
$\bar{X}$	arithmetic mean

Y	predicted response from a regression equation
z	standard score
(+)	significant
(–)	insignificant
(±)	possibly significant
↓	decreased, depression
↑	increased elevation
⇑	up
↑V	increase due to *in vivo* effect
↓V	decrease due to *in vivo* effect
↑C	increase due to chemical interference during assay
↓C	decrease due to chemical interference during assay
→	causes, no change, transfer to
←	is due to
⇌	reversible reaction
ϴ	normal
$\sqrt{c}$	check with
∨	systolic blood pressure
∧	diastolic blood pressure
#	gauge, number, weight, pound(s)
R_x	recipe, take
°	degree
24°	hours
1°	primary
2°	secondary
2d	second
2ndry	secondary
1×	once
2×	twice

×2	twice
Ⓛ	left
Ⓡ	right, trademark
Ⓜ	murmur
⊙	start of operation
⊗	end of operation
□	male
O	female
♂	male
O	female
*	birth
†	death
◡	combined with
Δ	prism diopter
Δt	time interval
ΔA	change in absorbance
Δ*p*H	change in *p*H
Ω	ohm
℥	ounce
f℥	fluid ounce
℈	scruple
♏	minim
ʒ	drachm, dram
ʒ	fluidrachm, fluidram
√	root, square root, radical
$\sqrt[2]{}$	square root
$\sqrt[3]{}$	cube root
:	ratio (is to)
: :	equality between ratios, "as"
∴	therefore
%	per cent
?	questionable, possible

Metric System Symbols

Symbol	*Name*	*Value*
T	tera	10^{12}
G	giga	10^{9}
M	mega	10^{6}
my	myria	10^{4}
k	kilo	10^{3}
h	hecto	10^{2}
dk	deka	10
d	deci	10^{-1}
c	centi	10^{-2}
m	milli	10^{-3}
μ	micro	10^{-6}
n	nano	10^{-9}
p	pico	10^{-12}
f	femto	10^{-15}
a	atto	10^{-18}

Greek Alphabet (letter and name)

Α	α	Alpha
Β	β	Beta
Γ	γ	Gamma
Δ	δ	Delta
Ε	ε	Epsilon
Ζ	ζ	Zeta
Η	η	Eta
Θ	θ	Theta
Ι	ι	Iota
Κ	κ	Kappa
Λ	λ	Lambda
Μ	μ	Mu
Ν	ν	Nu
Ξ	ξ	Xi
Ο	ο	Omicron
Π	π	Pi
Ρ	ρ	Rho
Σ	σ	Sigma
Τ	τ	Tau
γ	υ	Upsilon
Φ	ϕ	Phi
Χ	χ	Chi
Ψ	ψ	Psi
Ω	ω	Omega

APPENDIX-II

ESSENTIAL FORMULAE

1. **Arithmetic Mean ($\bar{x}$) :** $\bar{x} = \frac{\Sigma x}{n}$

2. **Range :** Range = Highest Value – Lowest Value

3. **Standard Deviation (σ) :** $\sigma = \sqrt{\frac{\Sigma(x-\bar{x})^2}{n}}$

4. **Variance :** Variance = σ^2

5. **A Sample Proportion :** $\frac{\text{Number of occurrences}}{\text{Sample size}}$

   or $\bar{p} = \frac{x}{n}$

6. **Standard Score :** $z = \frac{\text{Value} - \text{Mean}}{\text{Standard deviation}} = \frac{\chi - \mu}{\sigma}$

7. **Standard Error of a Mean :** $\sigma_{\bar{x}} = \frac{\sigma}{\sqrt{n}}$

8. **Standard Error of a Proportion :** $\sigma_{\bar{p}} = \sqrt{\frac{pq}{n}}$

9. **Rank Correlation Coefficient (r_r) :** $r_r = 1 - \frac{6\Sigma d^2}{n(n^2-1)}$

10. **Chi-Square (χ^2) :** $\chi^2 = \Sigma \frac{(\text{Actual} - \text{Expected Value})}{\text{Expected Value}}$

    $= \Sigma \frac{f_0 - f_t}{f_t}$

11. *t*-Test (One Sample) : $t = \frac{\bar{x} - \mu}{S_{\bar{x}}}$

(Two Samples) : $t = \frac{\bar{x}_1 - \bar{x}_2}{S\bar{x} - \bar{x}_2}$

12. F Test :$F = \frac{\text{Between – Treatment Variance}}{\text{Within – Treatment Variance}} = \frac{SSA/(c-1)}{SSE/(n-c)}$

13. Sample Size for Estimation of a Population Mean :

$$n = \frac{z^2\sigma^2}{D^2}$$

14. Average Annual Rate of Change : $[(P_n / P_0)^{1/N} - 1] \times 100$

where P_n = Value in later time period
P_0 = Value in earlier time period
N = Number of years between the two time periods.

15. Formula for Population Projection : $P_1 = P_0\,(1 + r)_n$

where P_1 = Population estimate for the projected year
P_0 = Population in base year
r = Annual growth rate
n = Number of years

APPENDIX-III

RATES AND RATIOS OF SELECTED HEALTH CARE INDICATORS AND THEIR CALCULATION

III-A. Demographic Indicators

III-B. Health Status Indicators

III-C. Indicators of Health Care Provision

Coverage

Accessibility

1. Primary Health Care Centre
2. Hospital Outpatient Department
3. Hospital

Utilization

1. Primary Health Care Centre & OPD
2. Hospital
3. Bed

III-D. Indicators of Health Care Quality

III-E. Indicators of the Availability of Health Manpower

III-F. Manpower Productivity Indicators

III-G. Indicators of Health Care Costs

III-H. Functional Indicators

Personnel Management

Financial Management

Food Service

Medical Records

III-A. Demographic Indicators

1. Crude Birth Rate:

$$\frac{\text{Number of live births in a given year}}{\text{Mid year population of that year}} \times 1000$$

2. Crude Death Rate:

$$\frac{\text{Number of deaths in a given year}}{\text{Midyear population of that year}} \times 1000$$

3. General Fertility Rate:

$$\frac{\text{Number of live births in a year}}{\text{Midyear female population, aged 15-49 during the same year}} \times 1000$$

4. Specific Fertility Rate:

$$\frac{\text{Number of live births occurring to females of a specified age-group during a year}}{\text{Midyear female population of the specified age-group during the same year}} \times 1000$$

5. Fertility Ratio:

$$\frac{\text{Number of girls under 15 years of age}}{\text{Number of women in 15-49 age group}} \times 1000$$

6. Gross Reproduction Rate:

$$\frac{\text{Number of female children born to 1000 females of the 15-49 age group}}{1000}$$

7. Net Reproduction Rate:

$$\frac{\text{Number of female children born (and survived) to 1000 females of the 15-49 age-group}}{1000}$$

8. Growth Rate of Population (Natural Rate of Increase):

$$\frac{\text{Live births during the year} - \text{Deaths during the year}}{\text{Midyear population of that year}} \times 100$$

9. Net Migration Rate:

$$\frac{\text{Number of overseas arrivals in a given year} - \text{Number of overseas departures in the same year}}{\text{Midyear population of that year}} \times 1000$$

10. Induced Termination of Pregnancy Rate:

$$\frac{\text{Number of induced terminations occurring during a period}}{\text{Female population, aged 15-49 years}} \times 1000$$

11. Induced Termination of Pregnancy Ratio:

$$\frac{\text{Number of induced terminations occurring during a period}}{\text{Number of live births occurring during the same period}} \times 1000$$

III-B. Health Status Indicators

1. Percentage of Low Birth Weight:

$$\frac{\text{Live born babies with birth weight less than 2,500 g}}{\text{Total number of live born babies}} \times 100$$

2. Percentage of Low Weight for Age:

$$\frac{\text{Number of children with low weight for age}}{\text{Total number of children}} \times 100$$

3. Percentage of Low Height for Age:

$$\frac{\text{Number of children with low height for age}}{\text{Total number of children}} \times 100$$

4. Percentage of Low Weight for Height:

$$\frac{\text{Number of children with low weight for height}}{\text{Total number of children}} \times 100$$

5. Percentage of Small Upper Arm Circumference:

$$\frac{\text{Number of children with small upper arm circumference}}{\text{Total number of children}} \times 100$$

6. Infant Mortality Rate:

$$\frac{\text{Number of deaths under one year of age during a period}}{\text{Number of live births during the same period}} \times 1000$$

7. Infant Mortality Rate (weight-specific):

$$\frac{\text{Infant deaths among live births weighing 1000 g and over at birth}}{\text{Live births weighing 1000 g \& over}} \times 1000$$

8. Child Mortality Rate:

$$\frac{\text{Number of deaths of children aged 1-4 years during a year}}{\text{Total number of children aged 1-4 years at the middle of the year}} \times 1000$$

9. Under-5 Mortality Rate:

$$\frac{\text{Number of deaths under-5 years of age in a given year}}{\text{Total number of children under-5 years of age at the middle of the year}} \times 1000$$

10. Under-5 Proportionate Mortality:

$$\frac{\text{Number of deaths under-5 years of age in a given year}}{\text{Total number of deaths during the same year}} \times 1000$$

11. Life Expectancy:

$$\frac{\text{Total number of years a given birth cohort can be expected to live}}{\text{Number of children in the cohort}}$$

12. Maternal Mortality Rate:

$$\frac{\text{Number of maternal deaths (direct or indirect) during a period}}{\text{Number of live births during the same period}} \times 1000 \text{ or } 100{,}000$$

13. Direct Obstetric Mortality Ratio:

$$\frac{\text{Direct obstetric deaths only, during a given period}}{\text{Number of live births during the same period}} \times 100{,}000$$

14. Pregnancy-Related Mortality Ratio:

$$\frac{\text{Pregnancy-related deaths during a given period}}{\text{Number of live births during the same period}} \times 100{,}000$$

15. Foetal Death Rate:

$$\frac{\text{Number of foetal deaths for a period}}{\text{Total number of births (live births + foetal deaths) for the same period}} \times 1000$$

16. Foetal Deaths Rate (weight-specific):

$$\frac{\text{Number of foetal deaths weighing 1000 g and over for a period}}{\text{Total number of births (live births + foetal deaths) weighing 1000 g and over for the same period}} \times 1000$$

17. Foetal Death Ratio:

$$\frac{\text{Number of foetal deaths for a period}}{\text{Number of live births for the same period}} \times 1000$$

18. Early Neonatal Mortality Rate:

$$\frac{\text{Number of early neonatal deaths for a period}}{\text{Number of live births for the same period}} \times 1000$$

19. Early Neonatal Mortality Rate (weight-specific):

$$\frac{\text{Early neonatal deaths of infants weighing 1000 g and over at birth for a period}}{\text{Live births weighing 1000 g and over for the same period}} \times 1000$$

20. Perinatal Mortality Rate:

$$\frac{\text{Number of foetal deaths and early neonatal deaths during a given period}}{\text{Number of total births (live births + foetal deaths) during the same period}} \times 1000$$

21. Perinatal Mortality Rate (weight-specific):

$$\frac{\text{Foetal deaths weighing 1000 g and over + early neonatal deaths of infants weighing 1000 g or over at birth}}{\text{Number of total births (live births + foetal deaths) weighing 1000 g and over}} \times 1000$$

22. Perinatal Mortality Ratio:

$$\frac{\text{Number of foetal deaths and early neonatal deaths during a given period}}{\text{Number of live births during the same period}} \times 1000$$

23. Neonatal Mortality Rate:

$$\frac{\text{Number of neonatal deaths during a given period}}{\text{Number of live births during the same period}} \times 1000$$

24. Neonatal Mortality Rate (weight-specific) :

$$\frac{\text{Neonatal deaths of infants weighing 1000 g and over at birth}}{\text{Live births weighing 1000 g and over}} \times 1000$$

25. Disease-Specific Death Rate:

$$\frac{\text{Number of deaths from a specific disease during a given year}}{\text{Midyear population of that year}} \times 100{,}000$$

26. Age-Specific Death Rate:

$$\frac{\text{Number of deaths among residents of a specified age group in a given year}}{\text{Midyear population of residents of the same specified age group in that year}} \times 100{,}000$$

27. Sex-Specific Death Rate:

$$\frac{\text{Number of deaths among residents of a specified sex in a given year}}{\text{Midyear population of residents of the same sex in that year}} \times 100{,}000$$

28. Sex-Age Specific Death Rates:

$$\frac{\text{Number of deaths among residents of a specified sex and age group in a year}}{\text{Midyear population of residents of the same specified sex and age group in that year}} \times 1000$$

29. Sex-Age Disease-Specific Death Rate:

$$\frac{\text{Number of deaths from the specific disease which occurred to a given age and sex group during a given year}}{\text{Midyear population of the same age and sex group, of that year}} \times 100{,}000$$

30. Proportionate Mortality Rate (from a specific disease):

$$\frac{\text{Number of deaths from a specific disease in a given year}}{\text{Number of deaths from all causes in that year}} \times 100$$

31. Case Fatality Rate (usually expressed as a percentage):

$$\frac{\text{Number of deaths from a disease in a given period}}{\text{Number of diagnosed cases of that disease in the same period}} \times 100$$

32. Incidence Rate:

$$\frac{\text{Number of new cases of disease appearing in a specified period of time}}{\text{Number of persons exposed to risk during the same specified period of time}} \times 1000 \text{ or } 100{,}000$$

33. Point Prevalence Rate:

$$\frac{\text{Number of sick persons existing at a specific point of time}}{\text{Number of persons exposed to risk within the same specified point of time}} \times 1000 \text{ or } 100{,}000$$

34. Period Prevalence Rate:

$$\frac{\text{Number of cases of a disease (new and old) at any time within a specified period}}{\text{Number of persons exposed to risk within the same specified period}} \times 1000 \text{ or } 100{,}000$$

35. Secondary Attack Rate:

$$\frac{\text{Number of secondary cases in a period of time}}{\text{Number of susceptible persons during the same time}} \times 1000$$

36. Long-Term Disability Prevalence:

$$\frac{\text{Number of persons suffering from long-term disability}}{\text{Total number of persons investigated}} \times 1000$$

III -C. Indicators of the Provision of Health Care

COVERAGE

1. Percentage of Women Receiving Antenatal Care:

$$\frac{\text{Number of first antenatal contacts}}{\text{Number of expected births}} \times 100$$

2. Percentage of Women Receiving Delivery Care:

$$\frac{\text{Number of supervised deliveries}}{\text{Number of expected births}} \times 100$$

3. Annual Obstetric Coverage (in a community):

$$\frac{\text{Number of deliveries attended by a qualified midwife or obstetrician}}{\text{Expected number of deliveries during the year in a given community}} \times 100$$

4. Annnal Immunization Coverage:

$$\frac{\text{Number of children (of a specified age-group) immunized against specific diseases}}{\text{Number of children (of a specified age-group) at risk}} \times 100$$

5. Rubella Immunization Rate:

$$\frac{\text{Number of women aged 25-44 years who have been immunized against rubella}}{\text{Total number of women aged 25-44 years}} \times 100$$

6. Mammography Screening Rate:

$$\frac{\text{Number of women aged 40-64 years who have had a mammogram in the last 3 years}}{\text{Total number of women aged 40-64 years}} \times 100$$

7. Pap Smear Screening Rate:

$$\frac{\text{Number of women aged 25-64 years who have had a Pap smear test in the last 3 years}}{\text{Total number of women aged 25-64 years}} \times 100$$

ACCESSIBILITY

1. Primary Health Care Centre

(i) *Population Per Health Care Centre (PHC):*

$$\frac{\text{Number of population in the area in a given year}}{\text{Number of PHC centres in that area in the same year}}$$

(ii) *Average time a patient stays in PHC centre to get the service needed (Average Transit Time):*

$$\frac{\text{Total time (in minutes) stayed in PHC Centre}}{\text{Total number of patients}}$$

(iii) *Average Waiting Time Per Patient:*

$$\frac{\text{Total time (in minutes) stayed by all patients in the PHC Centre, waiting to see the doctor(s)}}{\text{Total number of patients}}$$

2. Hospital Outpatient Department

(i) *Population Per OPD Specialist:*

$$\frac{\text{Service Population}}{\text{Number of specialists}}$$

(ii) *Waiting Days Per Patient:*

$$\frac{\text{Number of days a patient waits to see the specialist}}{\text{Number of patients on the appointment list}}$$

3. Hospital

(i) *Bed/Population Index:*

$$\frac{\text{Total number of hospital beds available}}{\text{Number of population}} \times 1000$$

(ii) *Patients Waiting Admission:*

$$\frac{\text{Number of patients who have been put on the waiting list}}{\text{Number of patients who need admission}} \times 100$$

(iii) *Average Waiting Time Before Admission:*

$$\frac{\text{Total number of days stayed waiting admission by patients on the waiting list}}{\text{Number of patients on the waiting list}}$$

(iv) *Physicians-Bed Ratio:*

$$\frac{\text{Number of hospital beds available}}{\text{Number of physicians}}$$

(v) *Nurse-Bed Ratio:*

$$\frac{\text{Number of hospital beds available}}{\text{Number of nurses}}$$

(vi) *Surgical Beds/Operating-Theatre:*

$$\frac{\text{Number of surgical beds available}}{\text{Number of operating theatres}}$$

UTILIZATION

1. Primary Health Care Centre

(i) *Average Daily Number of Visits in a Year:*

$$\frac{\text{Number of visits to PHC Centre in a year}}{\text{Number of working days in the year}}$$

(ii) *Average Number of Visits Per Individual in the Community:*

$$\frac{\text{Total number of visits to PHC Centres in a year}}{\text{Midyear population of that year}}$$

(iii) *Average Daily Number of Visits Per PHC Physician:*

$$\frac{\text{Number of visits to PHC in a year}}{\text{Number of physicians} \times \text{Number of working days in the year}}$$

(iv) *Daily Encounter (Visit) Rate:*

$$\frac{\text{Total number of encounters (visits)}}{\text{Midyear population} \times \text{Number of working days in the year}}$$

(v) *Rate of Referral from PHC Centre to Hospital OPD:*

$$\frac{\text{Number of patients referred from PHC physician to OPD}}{\text{Total number of visits to PHC physician}} \times 100$$

(vi) *Rate of Referral from OPD to Hospital:*

$$\frac{\text{Number of patients referred from OPD to hospital for admission}}{\text{Total number of visits to OPD specialist}} \times 100$$

(vii) *Rate of Referral by Physicians to Lab. Investigations:*

$$\frac{\text{Number of patients referred by OPD physicians to the Lab}}{\text{Total number of visits to physicians}} \times 100$$

(viii) *Rate of Referral by Physicians to X-ray Examinations:*

$$\frac{\text{Number of patients referred by OPD physicians to X-ray department}}{\text{Total number of visits to physicians}} \times 100$$

(ix) *Average Daily Number of Patients Per Specialist at the Outpatient Clinic:*

$$\frac{\text{Number of visits to a specialized outpatient clinic in a year}}{\text{Number of specialists} \times \text{Number of working days in the year}}$$

2. Hospital

(i) *Annual Hospital Discharge Rate:*

$$\frac{\text{Number of hospital discharges}}{\text{Number of population served}} \times 1000$$

(ii) *Annual Hospital Days of Care:*

$$\frac{\text{Number of hospital days of care provided}}{\text{Number of population served}} \times 1000$$

(iii) *Average Daily Inpatient Census:*

$$\frac{\text{Total inpatient service days for a period (excluding newborn)}}{\text{Total number of days in the period}}$$

(iv) *Average Daily Census for a Specific Care Unit:*

$$\frac{\text{Total service days for the unit for a period}}{\text{Total number of days in the period}}$$

(v) *Average Daily Newborn Inpatient Census:*

$$\frac{\text{Total newborn inpatient service days for a period}}{\text{Total number of days in the period}}$$

(vi) *Population/Health Personnel Ratio (Doctors, Dentists, Nurses, Pharmacists, etc.):*

$$\frac{\text{Number of population served}}{\text{Number of health personnel of the specified type}}$$

3. Bed

(i) *Bed Occupancy Rate:*

$$\frac{\text{Total service days for a period}}{\text{Total bed count days in the period}} \times 100$$

(ii) *Constant Vacancy Rate:*

100 – Highest occupancy rate

(iii) *Total Vacancy Rate:*

100 – Average occupancy rate

(iv) *Variable Vacancy Rate:*

Highest occupancy rate – Average occupancy rate

(v) *Lowest Occupancy Rate:*

$$\frac{\text{Lowest value of the daily census}}{\text{Beds available}}$$

(vi) *Highest Occupancy Rate:*

$$\frac{\text{Highest value of the daily census}}{\text{Beds available}}$$

(vii) *Bed Overload Rate:*

$$\frac{\text{Number of days beds were 100\% occupied in a year}}{365} \times 1000$$

(viii) *Average Length of Stay:*

$$\frac{\text{Total length of stay (days of care provided)}}{\text{Total discharges (including deaths)}}$$

(ix) *Bed Turnover Interval:*

$$\frac{\text{Total number of vacant days during a year}}{\text{Total discharges (including deaths) during that year}}$$

(x) *Bed Turnover Rate:*

Direct Formula:

$$\frac{\text{Number of discharges (including deaths) during a period}}{\text{Average bed count during that period}}$$

Indirect Formula:

$$\frac{\text{Occupancy Rate} \times \text{Number of days in a period}}{\text{Average length of stay}}$$

(xi) *Bed Need:*

$$\frac{\text{Average daily census}}{\text{Desired utilization rate}}$$

III-D. Indicators of the Quality of Health Services

1. Readmission Rate for the Same Condition Within One Month:

$$\frac{\text{Number of readmissions for the same condition within one month}}{\text{Total number of admissions during that month}} \times 100$$

2. Hospital Infection Rate:

$$\frac{\text{Number of infections among patients during a period}}{\text{Number of patients at risk of infection during that period}} \times 100$$

3. Surgical Operation Rate:

$$\frac{\text{Number of surgical operations}}{\text{Total number of hospital discharges}} \times 100$$

4. Post-operative Wound Infection Rate:

$$\frac{\text{Number of surgical wound infections}}{\text{Total number of surgical operations}} \times 100$$

5. Caesarean Section Rate:

$$\frac{\text{Total number of caesarean sections performed in a period}}{\text{Total number of deliveries in the period, including caesarean sections}} \times 100$$

6. Hospital Death Rate:

Gross Death Rate:

$$\frac{\text{Number of deaths of inpatients in a period}}{\text{Number of discharges (including deaths) in the same period}} \times 100$$

Net Death Rate :

$$\frac{\text{Number of deaths of inpatients in a period} - \text{Deaths occurring under 48 hours of admission}}{\text{Total number of discharges (including deaths)} - \text{Deaths under 48 hours of admission}} \times 1000$$

7. Hospital Maternal Mortality Rate:

$$\frac{\text{Number of maternal deaths in the hospital}}{\text{Number of hospital deliveries}} \times 100$$

8. Hospital Neonatal Mortality Rate:

$$\frac{\text{Number of neonatal deaths in the hospital}}{\text{Number of hospital deliveries}} \times 100$$

9. Anaesthesia Death Rate:

$$\frac{\text{Anaesthetic deaths for a period}}{\text{Number of anaesthetics administered for the period}} \times 100$$

10. Post-operative Death Rate:

$$\frac{\text{Deaths within 10 days after surgery}}{\text{Total number of operations performed during the period}} \times 100$$

11. Gross Autopsy Rate:

$$\frac{\text{Total inpatient autopsies for a given period}}{\text{Total inpatient deaths for the same period}} \times 100$$

12. Net Autopsy Rate:

$$\frac{\text{Total inpatient autopsies for a given period}}{\text{Total inpatient deaths – Unautopsied coroners' or medical examiners' cases}} \times 100$$

13. Complaint Rate Against Clinical Staff:

$$\frac{\text{Number of complaints against clinical staff}}{\text{Number of admissions}} \times 100$$

III- E. Indicators Pertaining to the Availability of Health Manpower

1. Per cent of Needed Positions Authorized:

$$\frac{\text{Number of authorized positions for a given year}}{\text{Number of needed positions for that year}} \times 100$$

2. Per cent of Authorized Positions Filled:

$$\frac{\text{Number of positions filled in a given year}}{\text{Number of authorized positions for that year}} \times 100$$

3. Manpower Turnover Rate:

$$\frac{\text{Number of persons lost in a given year (through firing, retirement, resignation or death)}}{\text{Mean number of persons in work during that year}} \times 100$$

III-F. Manpower Productivity Indicators

1. Surgical Operations Per Surgeon Per Year:

$$\frac{\text{Total number of surgical operations performed in a year}}{\text{Mean number of surgeons in that year}}$$

2. Surgical Operations Per Operating Room Per Day:

$$\frac{\text{Total number of surgical operations performed in a year}}{\text{Number of days in the year} \times \text{Number of operating rooms}}$$

3. X-ray Examinations Per Technician Per Day:

$$\frac{\text{Number of X-ray examinations performed in a year}}{\text{Number of X-ray technicians} \times \text{Number of days in a year}}$$

4. Laboratory Tests Per Technician Per Day:

$$\frac{\text{Number of lab tests performed in a year}}{\text{Number of laboratory technicians} \times \text{Number of days in the year}}$$

5. X-ray Examinations Per Patient:

$$\frac{\text{Number of X-ray examinations performed in a year}}{\text{Number of discharges and deaths in that year}}$$

6. Lab Tests Per Patient:

$$\frac{\text{Number of laboratory tests performed in a year}}{\text{Number of discharges and deaths in that year}}$$

7. Facility Utilization for Laboratory and Radiology:

$$\frac{\text{Hours of operation} \times \text{Days of operation}}{365 \times 24} \times 100$$

III-G. Indicators of Health Care Costs

1. Per cent of Government Expenditure on Health Services to Total Governmental Expenditure:

$$\frac{\text{Government expenditure on health services}}{\text{Total government expenditure}} \times 100$$

2. Per cent of Annual Increase in Governmental Expenditure on Health Services:

$$\frac{\text{Expenditure last year— Expenditure this year}}{\text{Expenditure last year}} \times 100$$

3. Per Capita Health Care Cost:

$$\frac{\text{Govemment expenditure on health care}}{\text{Number of population served}}$$

4. Per Capita Cost for Primary Health Care (PHC):

$$\frac{\text{Total PHC operating costs}}{\text{Number of population served}}$$

5. Cost Per Primary Health Care Visit:

$$\frac{\text{Total PHC operating costs}}{\text{Total number of PHC visits}}$$

6. Per Capita Outpatient Care Costs:

$$\frac{\text{Total outpatient costs of operation}}{\text{Total number of population served}}$$

7. Cost Per Outpatient Visit:

$$\frac{\text{Total outpatient cost of operation}}{\text{Total number of outpatient visits}}$$

8. Per Capita Inpatient Cost:

$$\frac{\text{Total hospital running costs (excluding outpatient costs and costs of emergency department)}}{\text{Number of population served}}$$

9. Inpatient Cost Per Case:

$$\frac{\text{Total hospital running costs (excluding outpatient costs and costs of emergency department)}}{\text{Total number of hospital discharges}}$$

10. Inpatient Cost Per Patient Day:

$$\frac{\text{Total hospital running costs (excluding outpatient costs and costs of emergency department)}}{\text{Total number of patient days}}$$

11. Construction Cost Per Hospital Bed:

$$\frac{\text{Total hospital construction costs}}{\text{Number of beds}}$$

12. Cost Containment:

$$\frac{\text{Cost savings + Cost avoidance}}{\text{Total operating costs}}$$

13. Breakeven Occupancy:

Per cent occupancy where revenue = Expense for running the health care facility

III-H. Functional Indicators

PERSONNEL MANAGEMENT

1. Grievance Rate:

$$\frac{\text{Number of grievances}}{\text{Mean personnel strength}}$$

2. Development Rate:

$$\frac{\text{Persons trained in service}}{\text{Mean personnel strength}}$$

3. Upgrading Rate:

$$\frac{\text{Persons upgraded}}{\text{Mean personnel strength}}$$

4. Overtime Rate:

$$\frac{\text{Overtime manhours}}{\text{Total manhours}}$$

FINANCIAL MANAGEMENT

1. Accuracy in Financial Forecasting:

$$\frac{\text{Budgeted staffing (or revenue, or expenditures)}}{\text{Actual staffing (or revenue, or expenditures)}}$$

2. Current Financial Ratio:

$$\frac{\text{Current assets}}{\text{Current liabilities}}$$

3. Debt Ratio:

$$\frac{\text{Total debt}}{\text{Total assets}}$$

4. Financial Coverage:

$$\frac{\text{Net income + Depreciation}}{\text{Interest and principal on debt}}$$

5. Financial Turnover:

$$\frac{\text{Patient revenue}}{\text{Total assets}}$$

6. Operating Margin:

$$\frac{\text{Net patient revenue}}{\text{Gross patient revenue}}$$

LOGISTICS MANAGEMENT

1. Supply Service Level:

$$\frac{\text{Requisitions filled}}{\text{Requisitions submitted}}$$

2. Equipment Replacement Level:

$$\frac{\text{Replacement expense}}{\text{Monetary value of items in use}} \times 100$$

3. Per cent of Equipment Inoperable:

$$\frac{\text{Items awaiting repair}}{\text{Number of items in use}} \times 100$$

4. Supply Turnover:

$$\frac{\text{Cost of supplies used}}{\text{Average inventory}}$$

5. Depreciation Rate:

$$\frac{\text{Annual depreciation}}{\text{Monetary value of plant and equipment in use}} \times 100$$

FOOD SERVICES

1. Patient Satisfaction:

$$\frac{\text{Number of complaints}}{\text{Meals served}} \times 100$$

2. Sanitation:

$$\frac{\text{Sanitation criteria met}}{\text{Sanitation criteria that should be met}} \times 100$$

3. Nutritional Adequacy:

$$\frac{\text{Daily nutritional requirements met}}{\text{Daily nutritional requirements that should be met}} \times 100$$

4. Efficiency:

(a) Manhours/meal served
Cost/meal served

(b) $$\frac{\text{Kilograms of edible waste}}{\text{Total kilograms of food served}} \times 100$$

MEDICAL RECORDS

1. Records Outstanding:

$$\frac{\text{Number of records incomplete}}{\text{Number of discharges}} \times 100$$

2. Records Lacking Diagnosis:

$$\frac{\text{Records lacking diagnosis}}{\text{Monthly discharges}} \times 100$$

3. Efficiency:

Manhours/discharge
Cost/discharge

4. Quality of Service:

$$\frac{\text{Number of professional criteria met}}{\text{Number of professional criteria that should be met}} \times 100$$

APPENDIX-IV

IMPORTANT HEALTH CARE ABBREVIATIONS

Abbreviation	Full Form
A&A	aid and attendance
A.A.	alcoholics anonymous
A.F.	atrial fibrillation, anal fissure, anal fistula
A.P.H.	ante-partum haemorrhage
A.P.N.	acute pyelonephritis
A.R.	allergic rhinitis, artificial respiration
A.S.	aortic stenosis, anxiety state
A.S.D.	atrial septal defect
A.S.R.	age standardized rate
A.C.T.H.	adrenocorticotropic hormone
A.D.H.	antidiuretic hormone
A.D.P.	adenosine diphosphate
A.L.N.	alanine aminotransferase (formerly S.G.P.T.)
A.P.M.	anterior poliomyelitis
A.S.T.	aspartate aminotransferase (formerly S.G.O.T.)
A.T.P.	adenosine triphosphate
B.A.	bronchial asthma, backache
B.A.C.	blood alcohol concentration
B.C.	birth control
B.C.G.	Bacille Calmette – Guerin (vaccine)
B.C.P.	birth control pill
b.d.	*bis die* (L), twice a day
B.I.	bone injury
B.M.I.	body mass index
B.M.R.	basal metabolic rate
B.P.	blood pressure
B.P.H.	benign prostate hypertrophy
Bx	biopsy
B.S.A.	body surface area
B.S.R.	basal sedimentation rate
B.U.N.	blood urea nitrogen
C.A.B.G.	coronary artery bypass graft

C&D	cystoscopy and dilatation
C.A.P.D.	continuous ambulatory peritoneal dialysis
C.A.T.	computerized axial tomography
C.H.D.	congenital/congestive/coronary heart disease
C.D.H.	congenital dislocation of the hip
C.H.F.	congestive heart failure
C.I.	confidence interval
C.N.S.	central nervous system
C.O.A.D.	chronic obstructive airways disease
C.O.D.	cause of death
C.O.I.	cost of illness
C.P.	cerebral palsy, chest pain, chronic pyelonephritis
C.P.I.	consumer price index
C.P.D.	cardio-pulmonary disease, cephalopelvic disproportion
C.R.F.	chronic renal failure
C.S.F.	cerebro-spinal fluid
C.S.O.M.	chronic suppurative otitis media
C.T.	cerebral thrombosis, coronary thrombosis, cerebral tumour
C.T. Scan	computed tomography scan
C.T.A.	chronic tonsillitis and adenitis
C.T.S.	carpel tunnel syndrome
C.V.A.	cardiovascular accident, cerebrovascular accident
C.V.D.	cardiovascular disease
C. V.S.	cardiovascular system, cardiovascular surgery
C.X.R.	chest X-ray
C	Celsius, centigrade, complement
C.B.C.	complete blood count
C.F.	complement fixation
Ci	Curie
C.K.	creatine kinase
C.P.R.	cardiopulmonary resuscitation
C.H.C.	community healthcare centre
D&C	dilatation and curettage (uterine)
D.L.E.	discoid/disseminated lupus erythematosus
D.M.	Diabetes mellitus, diabetic mother
dmft	decayed, missing or filled primary teeth
D.N.S.	deflected nasal septum

D.O.A.	dead on arrival
D.S.	Down's syndrome, disseminated sclerosis
D.T.	delirium tremens
D.U.	duodenal ulcer, diagnosis undetermined
D.U.B.	dysfunctional uterine bleeding
D.&V.	diarrhoea and vomiting
D.V.T.	deep vein thrombosis
Dx	diagnosis
D.X.T.	deep X-ray therapy
D.N.A.	deoxyribonucleic acid
D.T.P.	diphtheria-tetanus-pertussis (toxoids/vaccine)
D/W	dextrose in water
E.C.G.	electrocardiogram
Echo	echocardiogram, echoencephalogram
E.C.T.	electroconvulsive therapy
E.D.D.	expected date of delivery
E.E.G.	electroencephalogram
E.N.T.	ear, nose and throat
E.S.P.	extrasensory perception
E.S.R.	erythrocyte sedimentation rate
E.S.W.L.	extracorporeal shock wave lithotripsy
E.U.A.	examination under anaesthesia
Ez.	eczema
E.C.F.	extracellular fluid
E.F.R.	effective filtration rate
E.S.T.	electroshock therapy
F.B.	foreign body
F.D.I.U.	foetal death in utero
F.F.T.	free from infection, fever for investigation
F.T.I.	free thyroxine index
F.T.T.	failure to thrive
F.U.	follow-up, fractional urinalysis
F.U.O.	fever of unknown origin
fx	fracture, frozen section, fractional
F	Fahrenheit, Farad, female
F.D.A.	food and drug administration
F.H.R.	foetal heart rate

G.A.	gastric analysis, gestational age, general anaesthesia
G.D.P.	gross domestic product
G.I.	gastro-intestinal
G.P.	general practitioner
G.S.	general surgery
G.T.	glucose tolerance, group therapy
G.U.	gastric ulcer, genitourinary, gonococcal urethritis
gyn.	gynaecology
G.F.R.	glomerular filtration rate
G.R.	gamma ray, gastric resection
G.X.T.	graded exercise test
H.B.	heart block, hepatitis B
Hb.	haemoglobin
H.C.N.	health communication network
H.D.	herniated disc, heart disease, haemodialysis
H.D.L.	high density lipoprotein
H.E.W.	health, education and welfare
H.F.	hay fever, heart failure, high frequency
H.I.V.	human immunodeficiency virus
H.R.T.	hormone replacement therapy
H.V.	herpes virus, hallux valgus, hyperventilation
Hx	history
hy.	hysteria
H.Z.	herpes zoster
Hct.	haematocrit
H.I.	haemagglutination inhibition
H.L.A.	human leukocyte group A
Hz.	hertz (cycles/second)
I.B.S.	irritable bowel syndrome
I.C.U.	intensive care unit
I.D.	identification, infant deaths, infectious disease
I.D.D.M.	insulin-dependent diabetes mellitus
I.H.D.	ischaemic heart disease
I.I.D.M.	insulin-independent diabetes mellitus
I.M.	intramuscular, infectious mononucleosis, internal medicine
I.R.S.D.	index of relative socio-economic development

I.U.D.	intrauterine device, intrauterine death
I.V.	intravenous device, *in vitro, in vivo.*
I.V.F.	*in vitro* fertilization
I.V.P.	intravenous pyelogram
I.C.F.	intracellular fluid
I.C.P.	intracranial pressure
I.C.M.R.	Indian Council of Medical Research
I.D.K.	internal derangement of the knee joint
IgA	immunoglobulin A, etc.
I.O.F.B.	intraocular foreign body
I.S.Q.	*in status quo, i.e.* unchanged
I.U.R.	intrauterine growth rate
I.V.U.	intravenous urography
J.A.I.	juvenile amaurotic idiocy
jaund.	jaundice
JEE	Japanese equine encephalitis
JODM	juvenile onset Diabetes mellitus
J.R.A.	juvenile rheumatoid arthritis
J.V.	jugular vein, jugular venous
J.V.P.	jugular venous pulse
K.A.U.	King-Armstrong Units
K.F.D.	Kyasanur forest disease
K.M.V.	killed measles virus (vaccine)
K.U.B.	kidney, ureter and bladder
Kcal.	kilocalorie (food calorie)
k.j.	knee jerk
K.L.S.	kidney, liver, spleen
L.A.	local anaesthesia, left atrium, long-acting
L.B.	live births, loose body, low back
L.B.B.B.	left bundle branch block
L.B.P.	low back pain, low blood pressure
L.D.L.	low density lipoprotein
L.F.D.	low fat diet, low forceps delivery, least fatal dose
L.G.A.	large for gestational age
L.I.H.	left inguinal hernia
L.O.S.	length of stay, low output syndrome

L.&W.	living and well
L.D.H.	lactic dehydrogenase
L.E.	lupus erythematosus
L.B.W.	low birth weight
L.M.P.	last menstrual period, licenced medical practitioner
M.C.V.	mean cell volume, mean clinical value
M.I.	myocardial infarction, mitral incompetence
M.&N.	morning and night
M.O.H.	Medical Officer of Health
M.R.	mental retardation, mortality rate, mitral regurgitation
M.R.I.	magnetic resonance imaging
M.S.	multiple sclerosis, mitral stenosis
M.V.A.	motor vehicle accident
M.V.P.	mitral valve prolapse
My.	Myopia
M.	mega-, molar, thousand
M.C.H.	mean corpuscular haemoglobin, mother & child health (care)
M.C.H.C.	mean corpuscular haemoglobin concertration
M.S.W.	medical social worker, master of social work
mCi, mc	millicurie
M.I.C.	minimum inhibitory concentration
M.M.R.	measles, mumps, rubella, maternal mortality rate
N.A.D.	nothing abnormal detected
N.A.I.	non-accidental injury
N.B.W.	normal birth weight
N.D.	natural death, neonatal death, not done
N.D.I.	national death index
N.G.	new growth, nasogastric
N.I.D.D.M.	non-insulin-dependent diabetes mellitus
N.M.P.	normal menstrual period
N.N.D.	neonatal death
N.S.	nervous system, not significant, nephrotic syndrome
N.V.D.	nausea, vomiting and diarrhoea
N.Y.D.	not yet diagnosed
NSAID	nonsteroidal anti-inflammatory drug
N.S.S.	not statistically significant

N.T.P. normal temperature & pressure

O.A. old age, osteoarthritis
O.B.G. obstetrician-gynaecologist
O.C. on call, oral contraceptive
O.E.C.D. Organization for Economic Cooperation & Development
O.P.D. outpatient department
O.P.V. oral polio vaccine
O.R. operating room
O.T. occupational therapy, otolaryngology
O.T.C. over the counter
O.A.D. obstructive airway disease
O.B.P. ova, blood, and parasites
O.M. occupational medicine, osteomalacia, otitis media, osteomyelitis, occipitomental

Pap papanicolau
P.C.M. protein-calorie malnutrition
P.C.V. packed cell volume, polycythaemia vera
P.E. pulmonary embolism, physical examination
P.E.T. pre-eclamptic toxaemia
Pg. pregnant
P.H. public health, past history
P.I.D. prolapsed intervertebral disc, pelvic inflammatory disease
P.K.U. Phenylketonuria
P.M. post-mortem, preventive medicine
P.M.I.S. patient management information systems
P.O. postoperative
P.O.B. place of birth
P.O.D. place of death
P.P. postprandial, post-partum
P.P.H. postpartum haemorrhage
p.r. *per rectum* (L), through the rectum
P.U. peptic ulcer, pregnancy urine
P.V. *per vaginam* (L), through the vagina
P.X. physical examination
P.P.D. purified protein derivative

p.p.m.	parts per million
p.r.n.	*pro re nata* (as needed)
P.E.T.	positron emission tomography
P.H.C.	primary healthcare centre, posthospital care
Q.A.L.Y.	quality adjusted life year
Q.C.	quality control
q.d.	*quaque die* (L), every day
Q fever	query fever
q.h.	*quaque hora* (L), every hour
q.m.	*quaque mane* (L), every morning
q.n.	*quaque nocte* (L), every night
Q	quartile, quotient, volume of blood
quot	*quoties* (as often as necessary)
q.v.	*quantum vis* (as much as you please)
RA.	rheumatoid arthritis, radioactive
R.&D.	research and development
R.B.C.	red blood cell
R.D.I.	recommended dietary intake
R.D.S.	respiratory distress syndrome
R.E.	rectal examination, right eye
R.F.P.S.	risk factor prevalence study
Rh.	rhesus (factor)
R.I.H.	right inguinal hernia
R.R.	relative risk
R.T.	radiation therapy, radiotherapy, registered technician
R.T.A.	road traffic accident
Rx	prescription; *recipe* (L), take; treatment
R.F.	rheumatoid fever
R.N.A.	ribonucleic acid
S.&H.	speech and hearing
S.D.	septal defect, sudden death, spontaneous delivery
S.M.R.	standardized mortality ratio
S.O.B.	shortness of breath
S.O.S.	*si opus sit* (L), if necessary
S.S.	serum sickness, standard score, statistically

	significant
Sx	signs, symptoms
Syr.	*syrupus* (L), syrup.
SARS	severe acute respiratory syndrome
S.B.E.	subacute bacterial endocarditis
S.c.	subcutaneous (ly)
S.G.O.T.	serum glutamic oxaloacetic transaminase
S.G.P.T.	serum glutamic-pyruvic transaminase
S.I.	*Systeme International d' Unites* (International) System of Units)
S.L.E.	systemic lupus erythematosus
S.O.L.	space occupying lesion
S.T.S.	serological test for syphilis
S.T.D.	sexually transmitted disease
T&A	tonsils and adenoids, tonsillectomy and adenoidectomy
T.A.B.C.	typhoid and paratyphoid A, B & C vaccine
T.B.	tuberculosis, tubercle bacillus, tuberculin
T.B.L.C.	term birth, living child
T.D.	tetanus-diphtheria, typhoid dysentery, to deliver
t.d.	*ter die* (L), three times daily
T.P.R.	temperature, pulse and respiration
T.U.R.P.	transurethral resection of prostate
T.&X.	type and cross-match
T.V.H.	total vaginal hysterectomy
U.C.	ulcerative colitis, urea clearance, urinary catheter
U.G.	urogenital
U.R.T.I.	upper respiratory tract infection
U.T.I.	urinary tract infection
ux.	*uxor* (L), wife
U.V.R.	ultraviolet radiation
V.D.	venereal disease
V.E.	vaginal examination, visual efficiency
V.H.D.	valvular heart disease
V.S.D.	ventricular septal defect
V.S.O.K.	vital signs O.K. (normal)

V.V.	varicose veins, vulva and vagina
V&P	vagotomy and pyloroplasty
W.B.C.	white blood cell
W.C.	whooping cough, white cell, wheel-chair
W.H.R.	waist to hip ratio
W.H.O.	World Health Organization
W.H.R.C.	World Health Research Centre
W.L.	waiting list
W.R.	Wassermann reaction, weakly reactive
W.M.X.	whirlpool, massage, exercise
XOR	exclusive operating room
XR	X-ray
XX	normal female chromosome type
XY	normal male chromosome type
X.M.	crossmatch
Y.F.	yellow fever
Y.O.B.	year of birth
Y.A.G.	yttrium aluminum garnet (laser)
Z	zero, zone, standard score
Z/D	zero defects
Z.P.G.	zero population growth
Z.S.R.	zeta sedimentation ratio (method)

APPENDIX-V

COMBINING FORMS IN MEDICAL TERMINOLOGY

A. Some Components of Words Referring to Body Structure

Component	Pertaining to
aden-	glands(s), e.g. *adenoma*
angi-	vessels (esp. blood vessels), e.g. *angiography*
arthr-	joints(s), e.g. *arthritis*
aur-	ear(s), e.g. *auriscope*
broncho-	bronchi, lungs, e.g. *bronchitis*
cardi-	heart, e.g. *cardiologist*
caud-	lower part of the human body, e.g. *caudal*
cephal-	head, e.g. *cephalopathy*
cholangi-	bile ducts, e.g. *cholangitis*
chole-	biliary system, e.g. *cholesterol*
cholecyst-	gall bladder, e.g. *cholecystectomy*
chondr-	cartilage, e.g. *chondrosarcoma*
col-	colon, e.g. *colitis*
crani-	skull, e.g. *cranioplasty*
cyst-	bladder (esp. urinary bladder), e.g. *cystoscope*
dactyl-	finger(s), e.g. *dactylology*
dent-	tooth, teeth, e.g. *dentistry, dental*
derm-	skin, e.g. *dermatology, dermatitis*
encephal-	brain, e.g. *encephalitis*
enter-	intestine, e.g. *enteritis*
gastr-	stomach, e.g. *gastrectomy*
gingiv-	gum, e.g. *gingivitis*
gloss-	tongue, e.g. *glossitis*
hepat-	liver, e.g. *hepatitis*
hyster-	uterus, e.g. *hysterectomy*
lingua-	tongue, e.g. *lingual*
mamm-, mast-	breast, e.g. *mammogram, mastalgia*
myo-	muscle, e.g. *myocardium*
nephr-	kidney(s) e.g. *nephritis, nephrology*
ocul-, ophthalm-	eye(s) e.g. *oculist, ophthalmology*

orchid-	testis, e.g. *orchiopexy*
or-	mouth, e.g. *oral cavity*
oste-	bone,(s) e.g. *osteoma*
ot-	ear(s) e.g. *otitis*
ren-	kidney(s), e.g. *renal vein*
rhin-	nose, e.g. *rhinitis, rhinoplasty*
spondyl-	vertebra(e), e.g. *spondylitis*

B. Prefixes Used to Form Most Medical Words

Prefixes	Sense in which used	Examples with Meanings
a-	absence of	*abiosis,* absence of life
ab-	away from	*abduct,* to draw away (from
ad-	towards	midline)
an-	absence of	*adduct,* to bring towards (midline)
ana-	apart	*anaemia,* absence of blood
andr-	male	*anatomy,* to cut apart
ante-	before	*androgens,* male hormones
anti-	opposed to, against	*antenatal,* before birth
		antibiotic, opposed to living organisms
		antitoxin, against toxin
audi-	to hear	*auditory,* related to hearing
auto-	self	*autopsy,* examination after death
bi-	two	*bilateral,* on both sides
(di-)	two	*dioxide,* two oxides
bio-	life	*biopsy,* looking at living tissue
calc-	stone	*calculus,* stone formation in tissue
chrom-	colour	*chromosome,* coloured bodies in nucleus
con-	together with	*congenital,* "together with" (present) at birth
cyt-	cell	*cytoplasm,* plasma inside the cell
		cytology, study of the cell
demo-	people	*demography,* study of people (or populations)

dia-	through	*diarrhoea,* "flow through"
		diagnosis, "knowing through"
dis-	not,	*disease,* "not at ease" (ill)
	away	*dislocate,* "away from its place"
dys-	bad,	*dyspepsia,* "bad digestion"
	difficult	*dyspnoea,* "difficult breathing"
etc	outer,	*ectoderm,* "outer skin"
	out	*ectopic,* outside the uterus
end-	inner	*endoderm,* "inner skin"
	inside, in	*endoscope,* "instrument to look inside"
epi	upon	*epidermis,* "upon skin"
eu-	well, good	*euphoria,* "feeling good",
ex, exo	out,	*excision,* "to cut out"
extra	outside	*exophthalmos,* "bulging eyeballs"
		extrauterine, "outside the uterus"
gen-	birth,	*genitalia,* organs of reproduction
	reproduction	*genitourinary,* genital & urinary organs
gyn-	a woman	*gynaecology,* diseases of woman (study of)
haem-	blood	*haemorrhage,* "flow of blood"
		haemoglobin, a blood protein (globin)
hemi-	half	*hemiplegia,* paralysis of one side of body
hetero-	different	*heterogeneous,* of different kind or nature
homo-	same, alike	*homogeneous,* of the same kind or nature
hydro-	water, fluid	*hydrolysis,* breakdown by water
hyper-	above, in excess of	*hypertension,* abnormally high blood pressure
		hyperacidity, abnormally high acidity
hypo-	below, less than normal	*hypotension,* abnormally low blood pressure
		hypothermia, low body temperature

in-	in, not	*incision,* "a cutting in"
		inactive, not active
infra-	below	*infrared* "below red" (spectrum)
inter-	between	*intercellular,* between cells
intra-	within	*intracellular,* within cells
iso-	same, equal	*isomorphism,* sameness of form
lact-	milk	*lactose,* milk sugar
leuco-	white	*leucoderma,* "white skin"
(leuko)		*leukocyte,* white (blood) cell
lip-, lipo	fat	*lipoma,* cancer of fatty cells
lith-	stone	*lithiasis,* formation of stones in
macro-	large	the body
mal-	bad, faulty	*macrocyte,* a large blood cell
mega-	big	*malnutrition,* faulty nutrition
micro-	small	*megalocyte,* a large red blood cell
		microbiology, study of small
		living organisms
multi-	many	*multipara,* "many births"
myco-	fungus	*mycology,* study of fungi
para-	close to, near	*paranasal,* near the nose
peri-	around	*perinatal,* around birth
pneu-	air, lungs	*pneumonia,* inflammation of
		lungs
		pneumatic, pertaining to air or gas
poly-	many, much	*polyneuritis,* inflammation of
		many nerves
post-	after	*postnatal,* after birth
pre-	before	*prenatal,* before birth
pro-	before	*prognosis,* "knowing beforehand"
psych-	mind	*psychosis,* severe mental illness
py-, pyo-	pus	*pyuria,* pus in the urine
		pyorrhea, a discharge of pus
pyr-	fire, fever	*pyrexia,* fever
		pyrogen, fever inducing
		quadriplegia, paralysis of all 4
		limbs
quadri-	four	*tetravalent,* having a valency of
(tetra)	four	four

radio-	radiation	*radioactive,* emitting radiations
sub-	below	*sublingual,* below the tongue
supra-	above	*suprarenal,* above the kidneys
sym-	with	*symbiosis,* "living together"
syn-	union	*syndrome,* "to run together" (group of signs and symptoms that run together)
tox-	poison	*toxin,* a poisonous substance
tri-	three	*triplet,* 3 children at birth
ultra-	beyond	*ultrasound,* sound waves beyond the range of hearing
uni-	one	*unilateral,* one-sided
(mono-)		*monoplegia,* paralysis of one limb
vita-	life	*vital,* relating to life events

C. Suffixes Used to Form Most Medical Words

Suffix	Sense in which used	Examples with Meanings
-algia	pain	*myalgia,* painful muscles.
-ectomy	cutting out, removal	*appendicectomy,* removal of appendix.
-emia	a thing in blood	*uraemia,* urea and other nitrogenous products in blood.
-genic	producing	*pathogenic,* disease producing.
-graphy	recording	*radiography,* recording by X-rays.
-itis	inflammation	*dermatitis,* inflammation of skin.
-logy	study of	*cardiology,* study of heart and its diseases.
-lysis	breakdown	*hydrolysis,* breakdown with the help of water.
-myces	fungus	*actinomyces,* a species of fungi.
-natal	birth	*neonatal,* newly born.
-neo	new	*neoplasm,* new growth, cancer
-oma	tumour	*osteoma,* tumour of bone.
-osis	a condition of	*nephrosis,* a disease condition of kidney.
-ostomy	making an opening	*colostomy,* making an opening into the colon.
-otomy	cutting into	*tracheotomy,* cutting into the trachea.
-pathy	disease	*retinopathy,* disease of the retina.
-phil	loving	*eosinophilic,* "eosin-loving" (staining readily with eosin).
-phobe	fearing	*hydrophobia,* fear of drinking water.
-plegia	paralysis	*paraplegia,* paralysis of the lower part of the body including the legs.
-pnea	breath	*dyspnea,* difficulty in breathing.
-rrhea	flow, discharge	*diarrhea,* excessive flow of stools.
-rrhaphy	suturing	*herniorrhaphy,* suturing of hernia wound.
-scope	visual examination	*cystoscope,* instrument for looking at the bladder.
-uria	urine	*glycosuria,* sugar in urine.

APPENDIX-VI

LIST OF ESSENTIAL DRUGS

Note: Many drugs included in this list are preceded by an asterisk(*) to indicate that they represent an *example of a therapeutic group* and that various drugs could serve as alternatives. Example: **codeine:* other drugs for the symptomatic treatment of diarrhoea in adults, such as *loperamide* or, when indicated for treatment of cough, dextromethorphan.

1. Anaesthetics

1.1 General anaesthetics and oxygen

- diazepam
- ether, anaesthetic
- halothane
- ketamine
- nitrous oxide
- oxygen
- * thiopental

1.2 Local anaesthetics

- * bupivacaine
- * lidocaine

1.3 Preoperative medication

- atropine
- chloral hydrate
- * diazepam
- * morphine
- * promethazine

2. Analgesics, Antipyretics, Non-Steroidal Anti-Inflammatory Drugs

2.1 Non-opioids

- acetylsalicylic acid
- allopurinol
- colchicine

* ibuprofane
* indomethacin
* paracetamol

2.2 Opioid analgesics
* codeine
* morphine
  pethidine

3. Antiallergics and Drugs used in Anaphylaxis
* chlorpheniramine
* dexamethasone
  epinephrine
  hydrocortisone
* prednisolone

4. Antidotes and other Substances used in Poisonings

4.1 General
* charcoal, activated
  ipecacuanha

4.2 Specific
  atropine
  desferrioxamine
  dimercaprol
* methionine
  methylthioninium
  chloride
  (methylene blue)
  naloxone
  penicillamine
  potassium ferric
  hexacyanoferrate
  (II). $2H_2O$
  (Prussian blue)
  sodium calcium edetate
  sodium nitrite
  sodium thiosulfate

5. Antiepileptics

carbamazepine

* diazepam
phenobarbital
phenytoin
valproic acid

6. Anti-Infective Drugs

6.1 Anthelmintics
6.1.1 Intestinal
anthelmintics
levamisole
* mebendazole
piperazine
praziquantel
tiabendazole
6.1.2 Specific anthelminthics
albendazole
6.1.3. Antifilarials
diethylcarbamazine
ivermectin
suramin sodium
6.1.4 Antischistosomals
metrifonate
oxamniquine
praziquantel
6.2 Antibacterials
6.2.1 Penicillins
*amoxicillin
ampicillin
benzathine benzyl-penicillin
benzylpenicillin
*cloxacillin
phenoxymethylpenicillin
*piperacillin
procaine benzylpenicillin
6.2.2 Other antibacterials
*chloramphenicol
*erythromycin
*gentamicin

*metronidazole
spectinomycin
*sulfadimidine
*sulfamethoxazole + trimethoprim
*tetracycline
Complementary drugs
ciprofloxacin
clindamycin
doxycycline
nitrofurantoin
trimethoprim

6.2.3 Antileprosy drugs
clofazimine
dapsone
rifampicin

6.2.4 Antituberculosis drugs
ethambutol
isoniazid
pyrazinamide
rifampicin
rifampicin + isoniazid
streptomycin
Complementary drugs
thioacetazone +
isoniazid

6.3 Antifungal drugs
amphotericin
griseofulvin
* ketoconazole
nystatin
flucytocin

6.4 Antiprotozoal drugs

6.4.1 Antiamoebic and antigiardiasis drugs
* diloxanide
* metronidazole
chloroquine

6.4.2 Antileishmaniasis drugs
* meglumine antimoniate
pentamidine

6.4.3 Antimalarial drugs

(a) For curative treatment
 * chloroquine
 primaquine
 * quinine
 Complementary drugs
 mefloquine
 * sulfadoxine + pyrimethamine
 * tetracycline

(b) For prophylaxis
 chloroquine
 proguanil
 Complementary drug
 mefloquine

6.4.4 Antitrypanosomal drugs

(a) African trypanosomiasis
 melarsoprol
 pentamidine
 suramin sodium
 eflornithine

(b) American trypanosomiasis
 benznidazole
 nifurtimox

6.5 Insect repellents
 diethyltolumaide

7. Antimigraine Drugs

7.1 For treatment of acute attack
 acetylsalicylic acid
 ergotamine
 paracetamol

7.2 For prophylaxis
 * propranolol

8. Antineoplastic and Immunosuppressant Drugs and Drugs used in Palliative Care

8.1 Immunosuppressant drugs
 * azathioprine
 cyclosporine

8.2 Cytotoxic drugs
bleomycin
cisplatin
cyclophosphamide
cytarabine
dacarbazine
dactinomycin
* doxorubicin
etoposide
fluorouracil
mercaptopurine
methotrexate
procarbazine
vinblastine
calcium folinate

8.3 Hormones and antihormones
* dexamethasone
* ethinylestradiol
* prednisolone
tamoxifen

9. Antiparkinsonism Drugs

biperiden
levodopa + carbidopa

10. Drugs Affecting the Blood

10.1 Antianaemia drugs
ferrous salt
ferrous salt + folic acid
folic acid
hydroxocobalamin
* iron dextran

10.2 Drugs affecting coagulation
desmopressin
heparin
phytomenadione
protamine sulfate
* warfarin

11. Blood Products and Plasma Substitutes

11.1 Plasma substitutes
*dextran 70
* polygeline
11.2 Plasma fractions for specific uses
albumin, human
Complementary drugs
* factor VIII concentrate
* factor IX complex (coag. factors II, VII, IX, X) concentrate

12. Cardiovascular Drugs

12.1 Antianginal drugs
glyceryl trinitrate
*isosorbide dinitrate
* nifedipine
* propranolol
atenolol
12.2 Antidysrhythmic drugs
lidocaine
verapamil
atenolol
* procainamide
* quinidine
12.3 Antihypertensive drugs
* hydralazine
* hydrochlorothiazide
* nifedipine
* propranolol
Complementary drugs
atenolol
* captopril
methyldopa
* reserpine
* sodium nitroprusside
12.4 Cardiac glycosides digoxin
Complementary drug
digitoxin

12.5 Drugs used in vascular shock
dopamine
12.6 Antithrombotic drugs
acetylsalicylic acid
Complementary drug
streptokinase

13. Dermatological Drugs

13.1 Antifungal drugs (topical)
benzoic acid + salicylic acid
* miconazole
nystatin
sodium thiosulfate
Complementary drug
selenium sulfide
13.2 Anti-infective drugs
* methylrosanilinium chloride (gentian violet)
mupircoin
* neomycin + *bacitracin
silver sulfadiazine
13.3 Anti-inflammatory and antipruritic drugs
* betamethasone
* calamine lotion
* hydrocortisone
13.4 Astringent drugs
aluminium diacetate
13.5 Keratoplastic and keratolytic agents
benzoyl peroxide
coal tar
dithranol
fluorouracil
* podophyllum resin
salicylic acid
13.6 Scabicides and pediculicides
benzyl benzoate
permethrin
13.7 Ultraviolet-blocking agents
Complementary drugs

p-aminobenzoic acid, sun protection factor
* benzophenones, sun protection factor
* zinc oxide

14. Diagnostic Agents

14.1 Ophthalmic drugs
fluorescein
* tropicamide

14.2 Radiocontrast media
* amidotrizoate
barium sulfate
* iopanoic acid
* propyliodone
Complementary drug
* meglumine iotroxate

15. Disinfectants and Antiseptics

15.1 Antiseptics
* chlorhexidine
hydrogen peroxide
* iodine

15.2 Disinfectants
* calcium hypochlorite
glutaral

16. Diuretics

* amiloride
* furosemide
* hydrochlorothiazide
Complementary drugs
* mannitol
spironolactone

17. Gastrointestinal Drugs

17.1 Antacids and other antiulcer drugs

aluminium hydroxide
* cimetidine
magnesium hydroxide

17.2 Antiemetic drugs
metoclopramide
* promethazine

17.3 Antispasmodic drugs
* atropine

17.4 Anti-inflammatory drugs
hydrocortisone
sulfasalazine

17.5 Cathartic drugs
* senna

17.6 Drugs used in diarrhoea

17.6.1 Oral rehydration
Oral rehydration salts
(for glucose-electrolyte solution)

Components:	g/litre
sodium chloride	3.5
trisodium citrate dihydrate	2.9
potassium chloride	1.5
glucose	20.0

17.6.2 Antidiarrhoeal (symptomatic) drugs
* codeine

18. Hormones, other Endocrine Drugs and Contraceptives

18. 1 Adrenal hormones and synthetic substitutes
* dexamethasone
hydrocortisone
* prednisolone
fluorocortisone

18.2 Androgens
Complementary drug
testosterone

18.3 Contraceptives

18.3.1 Hormonal contraceptives

* ethinylestradiol + *levonorgestrel
* ethinylestradiol + *norethisterone
Complementary drugs
depot medroxyprogesterone acetate
* norethisterone

18.3.2 Intrauterine device
copper-containing device

18.3.3 Barrier methods
condoms with or without spermicide (nonoxinol)
diaphragms with spermicide (nonoxinol)

18.4 Estrogens
*ethinylestradiol

18.5 Insulins and other antidiabetic agents
insulin injection (soluble)
intermediate-acting insulin
* tolbutamide

18.6 Ovulation inducers
Complementary drug
* clomifene

18.7 Progestogens
norethisterone

18.8 Thyroid hormones and antithyroid drugs
levothyroxine
potassium iodide
* propylthiouracil

19. Immunologicals

19.1 Diagnostic agents
tuberculin, purified protein derivative (PPD)

19.2 Sera and immunoglobulins
anti-D immunoglobulin (human)
antiscorpion sera
* antitetanus immunoglobulin (human)
antivenom sera
diphtheria antitoxin

immunoglobulin, human normal
* rabies immunoglobulin

19.3 Vaccines

19.3.1 For universal immunization

BCG vaccine (dried)
diphtheria-pertussis-tetanus vaccine
diphtheria-tetanus vaccine
measles-mumps-rubella vaccine
measles vaccine
poliomylelitis vaccine (inactivated)
poliomyelitis vaccine (live attenuated)
tetanus vaccine

19.3.2 For specific groups of individuals

hepatitis B vaccine
influenza vaccine
meningococcal vaccine
rabies vaccine
rubella vaccine
typhoid vaccine
yellow fever vaccine

20. Muscle Relaxants (Peripherally Acting)

* gallamine
* neostigmine
suxamethonium

Complementary drugs

pyridostigmine
vecuronium bromide

21. Ophthalmological Preparations

21.1 Anti-infective agents

* gentamicin
* idoxuridine
silver nitrate
* tetracycline

21.2 Anti-inflammatory agents

* prednisolone

21.3 Local anaesthetics

* tetracaine

21.4 Miotics and antiglaucoma drugs

acetazolamide

* pilocarpine
* timolol

21.5 Mydriatics

atropine

epinephrine

22. Oxytocics and Antioxytocics

22.1 Oxytocics

* ergometrine oxytocin

22.2 Antioxytocics

* salbutamol

23. Psychotherapeutic Drugs

* amitriplyline
* chlorpromazine
* diazepam
* fluphenazine
* haloperidol

lithium carbonate

24. Drugs Acting on the Respiratory Tract

24.1 Antiasthmatic drugs

* aminophylline

beclometasone

epinephrine

* salbutamol

Complementary drugs

*cromoglycic acid

ephedrine

24.2 Antitussives

* codeine

25. Solutions Correcting Water, Electrolyte and Acid-base Disturbances

25.1 Oral rehydration
- Oral rehydration salts (for glucose-electrolyte solution)
- potassium chloride

25.2 Parenteral
- glucose
- glucose with NaCl
- potassium chloride
- sodium chloride
- sodium hydrogen carbonate
- * compound solution of sodium lactate

25.3 Miscellaneous
- water for injection

26. Vitamins and Minerals

- ergocalciferol
- iodine
- * nicotinamide pyridoxine
- * retinol
- riboflavin
- sodium fluoride
- thiamine

Complementary drugs
- ascorbic acid
- calcium gluconate

APPENDIX-VII

TRADE AND GENERIC NAME OF DRUGS

Generic Name	**Trade Name**
Acebutalol	SECTRAL
Acetaminophen	BATRIL, TYLENOL
Acetazolamide	DIAMOX
Acetohexamide	DYMELOR
Acetohydroxamic acid	LITHOSTAT
Acetophenazine	TINDAL
Acetylcysteine	MUCOMYST
ACTH	*See* CORTICOTROPIN
Acyclovir	ZOVIRAX
Adenosine	ADENOCARD
Albuterol	PROVENTIL, VENTOLIN
Allopurinol	ZYLOPRIM
Alprazolam	XANAX
Amantadine	SYMMETREL
Amikacin	AMIKIN
Amiloride	MIDAMORE
Aminocaproic acid	AMICAR
Aminophylline	SOMOPHYLLIN
Amiodarone	CORDARONE
Amitriptyline	ELAVIL, ENDEP
Amoxapine	ASENDIN
Amoxicillin	AMOXIL, LAROTID
Amphotericine B	FUNGIZONE
Ampicillin	AMCILL, OMNIPEN
Amrinone	INOCOR
Anisotropine	VALPIN
Anthralin	ANTHRA-DERM
Asparaginase	ELSPAR
Astemizole	HISMANAL
Atenolol	TENORMIN
Auranofin	RIDAURA
Azathioprine	IMURAN
Aziocillin	AZLIN
Aztreonam	AZACTAM
Baclofen	LIORESAL
Benzonatate	TESSALON
Benzquinamide	EMETE-CON
Benzoropine mesylate	COGENTIN
Beta carotene	SOLATENE
Betamethasone	CELESTONE, UTICORT

Generic Name	Trade Name
Betaxolol	BETOPTIC, KERLONE
Bethanechol chloride	DUVOID, URECHOLINE
Bisacodyl	DULCOLAX
Bitolterol	TORNALATE
Bleomycin	BLENOXANE
Bretylium	BRETYLOL
Bromocriptine	PARLODEL
Brompheniramine	DIMETANE
Bumetanide	BUMEX
Bupropion	WELLBUTRIN
Buspirone	BUSPAR
Busulfan	MYLERAN
Buterphanol	STADOL
Calcifediol	CALDEROL
Calcitonin-human	CIBACALCINE
Calcitonin-salmon	CALCIMAR
Calcitriol	ROCALTROL
Capreomycin	CAPASTAT
Captopril	CAPOTEN
Carbamazepine	TEGRETOL
Carbenicillin-i.s.	CEOPEN, PYOPEN
Carbidopa	SINEMET
Carbinoxamine	CLISTINE
Carboprost trom.	PROSTIN/15M
Carmustine	BICNU
Cefaclor	CECLOR
Cefadroxil	DURICEF, ULTRACE
Cefamandole	MANDOL
Cefazolin	ANCEF, KEFZOL
Cefixime	SUPRAX
Cefonicid	MONOCID
Cefoporazone	CEPHOBID
Ceforanide	PRECEF
Cefotaxime	CLAFORAN
Cefotetan	CEFOTAN
Cefoxitin	CEFOXITINE
Ceftazidime	FORTAZ, TAZICEF
Ceftizoxime	CEFIZOX
Ceftriaxone	ROCEPHIN
Cefuroxime	CEFTIN, ZINACEF
Cephalexine	KEFLEX
Cephapirin	CEFADYL
Cephradine	ANSPOR, VELOSEF
Chenodiol	CHENIX
Chloral hydrate	NOCTEC
Chlorambucil	LEUKERAN
Chloramphenicol	CHLOROMYCETIN

Generic Name	Trade Name
Chlordiazepoxide	LIBRIUM
Chlorhexidine	HIBICLEANS
Chlormezzanone	TRANCOPAL
Chlorotrianisine	TACE
Chlorpheniramine	TELDRIN
Chlorpromazine	THORAZINE
Chlorpropamide	DIABINESE
Chlorthalidone	HYGROTON
Cholestyramine	QUESTRAN
Cimetidine	TAGAMET
Ciprofloxacin	CEPTO
Cisplatin	PLATINOL
Clemastine	TAVIST
Clindamycin	CLEOCIN
Clofazimine	LAMPRENE
Clofibrate	ATROMID-S
Clomiphene	CLOMID
Clonazepam	KLONOPIN
Clonidene	CATAPRES
Clotrimazole	LOTRIMIN, MYCELEX
Cloxacillin	TEGOPEN
Clozapine	CLOZATIL
Colestipole	COLESTID
Corticotropin (ACTH)	ACTHAR
Cortisol	CORTEF, HYDROCORTONE
Cosyntropin	CORTROSYN
Co-trimaxazole	BACTRIM, SEPTRA
Cromolyn sodium	INTAL, NASALCROM
Cyclandelate	CYCLOSPASMOL
Cyclizine	MAREZINE
Cyclobenzaprine	FLEXERIL
Cyclopentolate	CYCLOGYL
Cyclophosphamide	CYTOXAN
Cycloserine	SEROMYCIN
Cyclosporine	SANDIMMUNE
Cyproheptadine	PERIACTIN
Cytarnbine	CYTOSAR-U
Dacarbazine	DTIC-DOME
Dactinomycin	DTIC-DOME
Dactinomycin	COSMEGEN
Danazol	DANOCRINE
Dantrolene	DANTRIUM
Daunorubicin	CERUBIDINE
Deferoxamine	DESFERAL
Demeclocycline	DECLOMYCIN
Desipramine	NORPRAMIN, PERTOFRANE
Desmopressin	DDAVP

Generic Name	Trade Name
Dexamethasone	DECADRON, HEXADROL
Dexchlorpheniramine	POLARMINE
Dextromethorphan	DELSYM, BENYLIN DM
Diazepam	VALIUM
Deazoxide, IV	HYPERSTATE
Deazoxide, oral	PROGLYCEM
Diclofenac sodium	VOLTAREN
Dicloxacillin	DYNAPEN, DYCILL
Dicyclomine	DENTYL
Diethylpropion	TENUATE, TEPANIL
Diflunisal	DOLOBID
Digitoxin	CRYSTODIGIN, PURODIGIN
Digoxin	LANOXIN
Dihydrotachysterol	HYTAKEROL
Diltiazem	CARDIZEM
Dimercaprol	BAL
Dinoprost	PROSTIN F2 ALPHA
Dinoprostone	PROSTIN E2
Diphenhydramine	BENADRYL
Diphenidol	VONTROL
Dipivefrin	PROPINE
Dipyridaole	PERSANTINE
Dissopyramide	NORPACE
Disulfiram	ANTABUSE
Divalproex	DEPAKOTE
Dobutamine	DOBUTREX
Docusate sodium	COLACE
Dopamine	INTROPIN
Doxepin	ADAPIN, SINEQUAN
Doxorubicin	ADRIAMYCIN
Doxycycline	VIBRAMYCIN
Dronabinol	MARINOL
Droperidol	INAPSINE
Edrophonium	TENSILON
Enalapril	VASOTEC
Encainide	ENKAID
Epoetin alfa	EPOGEN
Ergocalciferol	DELTALIN, DRISDOL
Erythromycin	ERYTHROCIN, E-MYCINE
Esmolol	BREVIBLOC
Ethacrynic acid	EDECRIN
Ethambutol	MYAMBUTOL
Etidronate sodium	DIDRONEL
Etoposide	VEPESID
Etrenate	TEGISON
Factor IX complex	KONYNE, PRPLEX
Famotidine	PEPCID

Generic Name	Trade Name
Fenfluramine	PONDIMIN
Fenoprofen	NALFON
Fentanyl	SUBLIMAZE
Flecainide	TAMBOCOR
Fluconazole	DIFLUCON
Flucystosine	ANCOBON
Fludrocortisone	FLORINEF
Flumethasone pivalate	LOCORTEN
Flunisolide	LIDEX
Fluoxetine	PROZAC
Fluoxymesterone	HALOTESTIN, ORATESTRYL
Fluphenazine	PERMITIL, PROLIXIN
Flurandrenolide	CORDRAN
Flurazepam	DALMANE
Flurbiprofen	ANSAID, OCUFEN
Furosemide	LASIX
Ganciclovir	CYTOVENE
Gemfibrozil	LOPID
Gentamicin	GARAMYCIN
Glipizide	GLUCOTROL
Glyburide	DIABETA, MECRONASE
Griseofulvin	GRIFULVIN, FULVICIN
Gauaifenesin	HYTUSS, ROBITUSSIN
Guanethidine	ISMELIN
Halazepam	PAXIPAM
Haloperiodol	HALDOL
Haloprogin	HALOTEX
Hydralazine	APRESOSOLINE
Hydrochlorothiazide	ESIDRIX, ORETIC
Hydrocortisone	*See* CORTISOL
Hydromorphone	DILAUDID
Hydroquinone	ELDOQUIN, ELDOPAQUE
Hydrosychloroquine	PLAQUENIL
Hydrosyurea	HYDREA
Dydrosyzine	ATARAS, VISTARIL
Ibuprofen	MOTIN, RUFEN
Idoxuridine	DENDRID, HERPLEX
Ifofamide	LOZOL
Indomethacin	INDOCIN
Ipratropium bromide	ATROVENT
Iron dextran	IMEFRON
Isoetharine	BRONKOSOL
Isoniazid	INH, NYDRAZID
Isopropamide iodide	BARBID
Isoproterenol	ISUPREL
Isosorbide dinitrate	ISORDIL, SORBITRATE
Isotretinoin	ACCUTANE

Generic Name	Trade Name
Kanamycin	KANTREX
Ketoconazole	NIZORAL
Detoprofen	ORUDIS
Ketorolac	TORADOL
Labetalol	NORMODYNE, TRANDATE
Lactulose	CEPHULAC, CHRONULAC
Levallorphan	LORFAN
Levamisole	ERGAMISOL
Levodopa	DOPAR, LARDOPA
Levothyroxine (T_4)	SYNTROID
Lidocaine	XYLOCAINE
Lincomycin	LINCOCIN
Lindane	KWELL
Liothyronine (T_3)	CYTOMEL
Liotrix	EUTHROID, THYROLAR
Lisinopril	PRINIVIL
Lithum carbonate	LITHANE, LITHONATE
Lomustine	CeeNU
Loperamide	IMODIUM
Lorazepam	ATIVAN
Lovastatin	MEVACOR
Loxapine	LOXITANE
Lypressin	DIAPID
Mafenide	SULFAMYLON
Maprotiline	LUDIOMIL
Mazindol	MAZANOR, SANOREX
Mebendaxole	VERMOX
Mechlorethamine	MUSTARGEN
Meclizine	ANTIVERT, BONINE
Meclofenamate	MECLOMEN
Medrosyprogesterone	PROVERA
Mefenamic acid	PONSTEL
Megestrol acitate	MEGACE
Melphalan	ALKERAN
Menodiol	SYNKAYVITE
Menotropins	PERGONAL
Meperidine	DEMEROL
Mephenytoin	MESENTOIN
Meprobamate	EQUANIL, MILTOWN
Mercaptopurine	PURINETHOL
Mesalamine	ROWASA
Mesoridazine	SERENTIL
Metaproterenol	ALUPENT, METAPREL
Metaraminol	ARAMINE
Methadone	DOLOPHINE
Methamphetamine	DESOXYN
Methandrostenolone	DIANABOL

Generic Name	Trade Name
Methdilazine	TACARYL
Methicillin	STAPHCILLIN
Methimazole	TAPAZOLE
Methocarbamol	ROBAXIN
Methotrimeprazine	LEVOPROME
Methoxsalen	OXSORALEN
Methsuximide	CELONTIN
Methyldopa	ALDOMET
Methylphenidate	RITALIN
Methylprednisolone	MEDROL
Methyltestosterone	METANDREN, ORETON
Methysergide	SANSERT
Metoclopramide	REGLAN
Metolazone	DIULO,ZAROXOLYN
Metronidazole	FLAGYL
Metyrapone	METOPIRONE
Mexiletine	MEXITIL
Mezlocillin	MEZLIN
Miconazole	MICATIN, MONISTAT
Minocycline	MINOCIN
Minoxidil	LONTTEN
Misoprostol	CYTOTEC
Mitomycin	MUTAMYCIN
Mitotane	LYSODREN
Molindone	MOBAN
Moxalactam	MOXAM
Nadolol	CORGARD
Nafcillin	UNIPEN
Nalbuphine	NUBAIN
Nalidixic acid	NEGRAM
Naloxone	NARCAN
Naltrexone	TREXAN
Nandrolone	DURABOLON
Naproxen	NAPROSYN
Neostigmine	PROSTIGMIN
Niclosamide	NICLOCIDE
Nefedipine	PROCARDIA
Nimodipine	NIMOTOP
Nitrofurantoin	FURADANTIN, MACRODANTIN
Nitroprusside	NEPRIDE
Nazatidine	AXID
Norfloxacin	NOROXIN
Nortriptyline	AVANTYL
Nystatin	MYCOSTATIN, NILSTAT
Octreotide	SANDOSTATIN
Omeprazol	PRILOSEC
Oxacillin	BACTOCILL. PROSTAPHLIN

Generic Name	Trade Name
Oxamniquine	VANSIL
Oxandrolone	ANAVAR
Oxazepam	SERAX
Oxybutynin	DITROPAN
Oxymetazoline	AFRIN, DURATION
Oxymetolone	ANADROL
Oxytocin	PITOCIN, SYNTOCINON
Pancrelipase	COTAZYM, ILOZYME
Pancuronium	PAVULON
Papaverine	CERESPAN, PAVABID
Paramethadione	PARADIONE
Paramethasone	HALDRONE
Pargylin	EUTONYL
Paromomycin	HUMATIN
Penicillamine	CUPRIMINE
Penicillin G benzathine	BICILLIN, PERMAPEN
Penicillin G potassium	PENTIDS
Penicillin G procaine	DURACILLIN, WYCILLIN
Penicillin V	PEN-VEE, V-CILLIN
Pentazocine	TALWIN
Pentobarbital	NEMBUTAL
Pentoxifylline	TRENTAL
Pergolide	PERMAX
Perphenazine	TRILAFON
Phenacemide	PHENURONE
Phenazopyridine	PYRIDIUM
Phenelzine	TRILAFON
Phenmetrazine	PRELUDIN
Phenobarbital	LUMINAL
Phenoxybenzamine	DIBENZYLINE
Phensuximide	MILONTIN
Phentermine	IONAMIN
Phentolamine	REGITINE
Phenylbutazone	AZOLID, BUTAZOLIDIN
Phenylephrine	NEO-SYNEPHRINE
Phenytoin	DILANTIN
Phytonadione	KONANKION, MEPHYTON
Pindolol	VISKEN
Peperacillin	PIPRACIL
Piperazxine	ANTEPAR, BRYREL
Pipobroman	VERCYTE
Piroxicam	FELDINE
Plicamycin	MITHRACIN
Pralidoxime	PROTOPAM
Prazepam	CENTRAX
Praziquantel	BILTRICIDE
Prazocin	MINIPRESS

Generic Name	Trade Name
Prednisolone	DELTA-CORTEF, HYDELTRAS
Prednisone	DELTASONE, METICORTEN
Primidone	MYSOLINE
Probenecid	BENEMID
Probucol	LORELCO
Procainamide	PRONESTYL, PROCAN SR
Procain	NOVOCAIN
Procarbazine	MATULANE
Prochlorperazine	COMPAZINE
Procyclidine	KEMADRINE
Promazine	SPARINE
Promethazine	PHENERGAN
Propantheline	PRO-BANTINE
Proparacaine	OPHTHETIC, OPHTHAINE
Propiomazine	LARGON
Propoxyphene	DARVON, DOLENE
Propranolol	INDERAL
Protripttyline	VIVACTIL
Pseudoephedrine	SUDAFED
Pyrantel pamoate	ANTIMINTH
Pyridostigmine	MESTNON
Pyrimetamine	DARAPRIM
Pyrvinium pamoate	POVAN
Quinacrine	ATABRINE
Quinethazone	HYDROMOX
Quinidine	CARDIOQUIN, QUINORA
Ranitidine	ZANTAC
Ribavirin	VIRAZOLE
Rifampin	RIFADINE, RIMACTANE
Ritodrine	YOTOPAR
Secobarbital	SECONAL
Selenium sulfide	SELSUN
Sildenafil citrate	VIAGRA, PENAGRA
Silver sulfadiazine	SILVADENE
Simethicone	MYLICON, SILAIN
Somatrem	PROTROPIN
Somatropin	HUMATROPE
Spectinomycin	TROBICIN
Spironolactone	ALDACTONE
Stanozolol	WINSTROL
Streptokinase	KABIKINASE, STREPTAASE
Streptozocin	ZANOSAR
Sucralfate	CARAFATE
Sulfamethoxazole	GANTANOL
Sulfasalazine	AZULFIDINE
Sulfinpyrazone	ANTURANE
Sulfisoxazole	GANTRISIN

Generic Name	Trade Name
Sulindac	CLINORIL
Suprofen	PROFENAL
Tamoxifen	NOLVADEX
Temazepam	RESTORIL
Terbutaline	BRETHINE, BRICANYL
Terfenadine	SELDANE
Testolactone	TESLAC
Testosterone, c.	DEPO-TESTOSTERONE
Testosterone, e.	DELATESTRYL
Tetanus imm. Globulin	HYPER-TET
Tetracyclline	TETREX, TETRACYN, ACHROMYCIN
Theophyline	THEOPDUR, THEOPHYL, ELIXOPHYLLIN
Thiabendazole	MINTEZOL
Thiethylperazine	TORECAN
Thioridazine	MELLARIL
Thiothixene	NAVANE
Thyrotropin	THYTROPAR
Ticarcillin	TICAR
Timolol maleate	BLOCADREN, TIMOPTIC
Tobramycin	NEBSIN
Tocainide	TONOCARD
Tolazamide	TOLINASE
Tolazoline	PRISCOLINE
Tolbutamide	ORINASE
Tolmetin	TOLECTIN
Tolnaftate	TINACTIN
Tranylcypromine	PARNATE
Trazodone	DESYREL
Tretinoin	RETIN-A
Triacetin	ENZACTIN
Triamcinolone	ARISTOCORT, KENACORT, KENALOG
Triamterene	DYRENIUM
Triazolam	HALCYON
Triclofos	TRICLOS
Trientine	CUPRID
Trifluridine	VIROPTIC
Trifluoperazine	STELAZINE
Triflupromazine	VESPRIN
Trimethadione	TRIDIONE
Trimethaphan	ARFONAD
Trimethobenzamide	TIGAN
Trimethoprim	PROLOPRIM, TRIMPEX
Trimethoprim-sulfamethoxazole	COMOXOL, SEPTRA, BACTRIM.
Trimipramine	SUMONTIL

Generic Name	Trade Name
Tripelennamine	PBZ
Triprolidine	ACTIDIL
Tromethamine	THAM
Tropicamide	MYDRIACYL
Valproic acid	DEPAKENE
Vancomycin	VANCOCIN
Vasopressin	PITRESSIN
Verapamil	CALAN, ISOPTIN
Vadarabine	VIRA-A
Vinblastine	VELBAN
Vincristine	ONCOVIN
Warfarin	COUMADIN, PANWARFIN
Zidovudine	RETROVIR

APPENDIX-VIII

NORMAL CLINICAL VALUES

1. Normal Clinical Values in Conventional and S.I. Units

Constituents	Conventional	S.I. Units
Albumin, Serum	3.5-5.5 g/dL.	35-55g/L.
Ammonia, Blood	80-110 μg/dL.	47-65 μmol/L.
Amylase, Serum	80-180 S.U./dL.	0.8-3.2 IU/L.
Bicarbonate, Serum or Plasma	24-28 mEq/dL.	24-28 mmol/L.
Bilirubin, Serum	0.2-1.2 mg/dL.	3.5-20.5 μmol/L.
Blood Urea Nitrogen, Serum or Plasma	8-25 mg/dL.	2.9-8.9 mmol/L.
Calcium, Serum	4.2-5.2 mEq/L.	2.1-2.6 mmol/L.
Copper, Serum	100-200 μg/dL.	16-31 μmol/L.
Chloride, Serum or Plasma	96-106 mEq/L.	96-106 mmol/L.
Cholesterol, Serum or Plasma	150-280 mg/dL.	3.9-7.2 mmol/L.
CO Contents, Serum or Plasma	24-29 mEq/L.	24-29 mmol/L.
Creatinine, Serum or Plasma	0.7-1.5 mg/dL.	60-132 μmol/L.
Globulin, Serum or Plasma	2-3.6 g/dL.	20-36 g/L.
Glucose, Serum or Plasma	65-110 mg/dL.	3.6-6.1 mmol/L.
Iron, Serum	50-175 μg/L.	9-31.3 μmol/L.
Iron-Binding Capacity, Serum	250-410 μg/dL.	45-73 μmol/L.
Lipids, Total Serum	450-1000 mg/dL.	4.5-10 g/L.
Magnesium, Serum	1.5-2.5 mEq/L.	0.75-1.25 mmol/L.
Nonprotein Nitrogen (NPN)	15-35 mg/dL.	14-21 mmol/L.
Phosphorus, Inorganic, Serum	3-4.5 mg/dL.	1-1.5 mmol/L.
Potassium, Serum or Plasma	3.5-5 mEq/L.	3.5-5 mmol/L.
Pyruvate, Blood	0.6-1 mg/dL.	70-114 μmol/L.
Sodium, Serum or Plasma	136-145 mEq/L.	136-145 mmol/L.
Sulfate, Serum or Plasma	0.5-1.5 mg/dL.	156-468 μmol/L.
Thyroxine (T), Total, Serum	5-14 μg/dL.	64-180 nmol/L.
Thyroxine, free, Serum (FT)	0.8-2.4 ng/dL.	0.01-0.03 nmol/L.
Total Protein, Serum	6-8 g/dL.	60-80 g/L.
Triglycerides, Serum	<165 mg/dL.	<1.65 g/L.
Urea, Serum or Plasma	21-53 mg/dL.	3.5-8.8 mmol/L.
Uric Acid, Serum or Plasma	2.5-9 mg/dL.	0.15-0.45 mmol/L.

Constituents	Conventional	S.I. Units
Uric Acid, Urine	350-600 mg/24 hr.	2.1-3.6 mmnol/24hr.
Vitamin A, Serum	15-60 μg/dL.	0.53-2.1 μmol/L.
Vitamin B, Serum	>200 pg/mL.	>148 pmol/L.
Vitamin C, Plasma	0.4-1.5 mg/dL.	22.7-85.3 μmol/L.
Vitamin D, Serum	21-45 pg/mL.	16-40 pmol/L.
Zinc	50-150 μg/dL.	7.6-22.9 μmol/L.

2. Normal Haematologic Values

Determination	Conventional	S.I. Units
Haemoglobin	Male: 13-18 g/dL.	8.1-11.2 mmol/L.
	Female 12-16 g/dL.	7.4-9.9 mmol/L.
Leukocyte (WBC) Count	4300-10,800/μL.	$4.3\text{-}10.8 \times 10^9$/L.
Erythrocyte (RBC) Count	4.2-5.9 million/μL.	$4.2\text{-}5.9 \times 10^{12}$/L.
Platelet Count	150,000-350,000/μL.	$150\text{-}350 \times 10^9$/L.
Haematocrit	Male: 45-52%	0.45-0.52
	Female 37-48%	0.37-0.48
MCV (Mean Corp. Volume)	86-98 μm/cell	86-98 fl (femtolitre)
MCH (Mean Corp. Haemoglobin)	27-32 pg	1.7-2.0 pg/cell
MCHC (Mean Corp. Hb. Conc.)	32-36 %	0.32-0.36
ESR (Eryth. Sed. Rate)	Male: 1-13 mm/h	1-13 mm/h
	Female 1-20 mm/h	1-20mm/h
WBC Differential :		
Myelocytes	0%	
Juvenile neutrophils	0%	
Band neutrophils	0-5%	
Segmented neutrophils	40-60%	
Lymphocytes	20-40%	
Eosinophils	1-3%	
Basophils	0-1%	
Monocytes	4-8%	

3. Normal Cerebrospinal Fluid Values

Determination	Conventional	S.I. Units
Albumin	11-48 mg/dL.	0.11-0.48 g/L.
Chloride	120-130 mEq/L.	120-130 mmol/L.
Glucose	50-70 mg/dL.	2.8-4.2 mmol/L.

Determination	Conventional	S.I. Units
IgG	2-6 mg/dL.	0.02-0.06 g/L.
Protein		
Lumbar	15-45 mg/dL.	0.15-0.45 g/L.
Cisternal	15-25 mg/dL.	0.15-0.25 g/L.
Ventricular	5-15 mg/dL.	0.05-0.15 g/L.
Pressure		
Newborn	30-80 mm of water	
Children	50-100 mm of water	
Adult	70-180 mm of water	

APPENDIX-IX

COMMON TESTS AND THEIR DISEASE ASSOCIATIONS

Laboratory Test	***Increase***	***Decrease***
Acid phosphatase	Prostatic carcinoma, postprostatic massage, prostatitis, myocardial infarction, excess platelet destruction, bone disease, liver disease	
Alanine aminotransferase (ALT or SGPT)	Hepatitis, cirrhosis, liver metastases, obstructive jaundice, infectious mononucleosis hepatic congestion, pancreatitis, ethanol ingestion, renal disease	Pyridoxine (vitaming B_6) deficiency
Albumin	Dehydration, diabetes insipidus	Overhydration, malnutrition, malabsorption, hepatic failure, nephrosis, burns, multiple myeloma, metastatic carcinoma
Alkaline phosphatase	Bone growth, bone metastases, Paget's disease, rickets, healing fracture, hyperparathyroidism, obstructive jaundice, hepatic disease, hepatic metastases, pulmonary infarction, heart failure, pregnancy	Pernicious anaemia, hypoparathyroidism, hypophosphatasia

Laboratory Test	***Increase***	***Decrease***
Alpha (α) Faetoprotein	Hepatoma, testicular tumour, hepatitis	
Amylase	Pancreatitis, GI obstruction, mesenteric thrombosis and infarction, macroamylasemia, parotitis, mumps, renal disease, ruptured tubal pregnancy, lung carcinoma, post-operative abdominal surgery, acute ethanol ingestion	Marked pancreatic destruction
Aspartate aminotransferase (AST or SGOT)	Myocardial infarction, heart failure, myositis, myocarditis, pericarditis, muscular dystrophy, trauma, hepatic disease, pancreatitis, eclampsia, renal infarct, neoplasia, cerebral damage, seizures, haemolysis	Pyridoxine (vitamin B_6) deficiency, terminal stages of liver disease
Bilirubin	Hepatic disease, obstructive jaundice, Gilbert's disease, haemolytic anaemia, pulmonary infarct, Dubin-Johnson syndrome, neonatal jaundice	
Calcium	Hyperparathyroidism, bone metastases, myeloma, sarcoidosis, hyperthyroidism, malignancy without bone metastases, hypervitaminosis D, milk-alkali syndrome	Hypoparathyroidism, renal failure, malabsorption, pancreatitis, Vitamin D deficiency, hypoalbuminaria, overhydration

Laboratory Test	***Increase***	***Decrease***
Cholesterol	Hypothyroidism, obstructive jaundice, nephrosis, diabetes mellitus, pancreatitis, pregnancy, familial factors	Hyperthyroidism, infection, malnutrition, heart failure, malignancies, severe liver damage (due to chemicals, drugs, hepatitis)
HDL cholesterol	Vigorous exercise, increased clearance of triglycerides (VLDL), moderate ethanol consumption, insulin, estrogens	Starvation, obesity, cigarette smoking, diabetes mellitus, hypothyroidism, nephrosis, liver disease, uraemia
Creatine kinase	Myocardial infarction, muscle disease, burns, chest trauma, collagen-vascular disease, meningitis, drugs (*e.g.* lovastatin), brain infarction, status epilepticus, hyperthermia, postoperative increase	
Creatinine	Renal failure, urinary obstruction, muscle disease, dehydration, hyperthyroidism, diet	Aging
Glucose	Diabetes mellitus, IV glucose, thiazides, corticosteroids, pheochromocytoma, brain damage, hyperthyroidism, Cushing's syndrome, acromegaly, hepatic disease, haemochromatosis, nephrosis, stress (*e.g.* emotions, burns, shock,	Excess insulin, insulinoma, Addison's disease, myxedema, hepatic failure, malabsorption, pancreatitis, glucagon deficiency, extrapancreatic tumours, early diabetes mellitus, post gastrectomy, autonomic nervous system disorders, idiopathic leucine sensivity,

Laboratory Test	Increase	Decrease
	anaesthesia), acute or chronic pancreatitis, Wernicke's encephalopathy (Vitamin B_1 deficiency), ephinephrine, estrogens, ethanol, phenytoin, chronic hypervitaminosis A	enzyme diseaes (von Gierke's disease, fructose intolerance), oral hypoglycemic drugs, malnutritition, alcoholism
Lactate dehydrogenase (LDH)	Myocardial infarction, pulmonary infarction, haemolytic anaemia, leukemia, lymphoma, other maliganancies, hepatic disease, trauma, sprue, renal infarction, seizures, cerebral damage	
Lipase	Same as amylase (except not in parotitis, mumps, macroamylasemia)	
Magnesium	Renal disease, excess Mg (IV or po)	Diarrhoea, malabsorption, renal tubular acidosis, acute tubular necrosis, chronic glomerulo-nephritis, drugs (diuretics, antibiotics), aldosteronism, hyperthyroidism, hypercalcemia, uncontrolled diabetes, nutritional deficit
Phosphorus	Renal failure, hypoparathyroidism, diabetic acidosis, acromegaly, hyperthyroidism, high phosphate intake	Hyperparathyroidism, osteomalacia, Fanconi's syndrome, rickets, cirrhosis, hypokalemia, excess IV glucose,

Laboratory Test	*Increase*	*Decrease*
	(IV or po), Vitamin D intoxication, lactic acidosis, cell lysis, leukemia, volume contraction, hyperlipidemia, hyperbilirubinemia, dysproteinemia	respiratory alkalosis, dietary deprivation, alcoholism, gout, haemodialysis
Potassium	Hyperkalemic acidosis, diabetic acidosis, hypoadrenalism, hereditary hyperkalemia, haemolysis, myoglobinuria, renal tubular defect, thrombocytosis, ACE inhibitors	Cirrhosis, malnutrition, vomiting, metabolic alkalosis, diarrhea, nephrosis, hyperadrenalism, diuretics, familial periodic paralysis, ectopic ACTH excess, β -hydroxylase deficiency
Sodium	Dehydration, diabetes insipidus, excessive salt ingestion, diabetes mellitus with diuresis, diuretic phase of acute tubular necrosis, hypercalcemic nephropathy with diuresis, "essential" hypernatremia due to hypothalamic lesions	Excess antidiuretic hormone, nephrosis, hypoadrenalism,myxedema, heart failure, diarrhea, vomiting, diabetic acidosis, diuretics, adrenocortical insufficiency, hyperlipidemia, mannitol, hyperglycemia, hyperproteinuria (*e.g.* multiple myeloma)
Total protein	Multiple myeloma, myxedema, sarcoidosis, lupus, dehydration, diabetes insipidus, collagen disease	Burns, cirrhosis, malnutrition, malabsorption, overhydration, GI protein loss
Triglyceride	Nephrosis, cholestasis, pancreatitis, diabetes mellitus, cirrhosis, hepatitis, hereditary, dietary excess	Malnutrition

Laboratory Test	*Increase*	*Decrease*
Urea nitrogen	Renal disease, dehydration, GI bleeding, leukemia, heart failure, shock, postrenal azotemia, any obstruction of urinary tract (BUN : creatinine > 10:1) acute myocardial infarction	Hepatic failure, overhydration, pregnancy, diet, acromegaly, IV feedings only
Uric acid	Gout, renal failure, diuretic therapy, leukemia, lymphoma, polycythemia, acidosis, psoriasis, hypothyroidism, eclampsia, multiple myeloma, pernicious anaemia, tissue necrosis, inflammation, cancer chemotherapy, haemolytic anaemia, sickle cell anaemia, high protein weight-reduction diet, lead poisoning, Lesch-Nyhan syndrome, polycystic kidneys, hypoparathyoridism, elevated serum triglycerides, sarcoidosis	Uricosuric drugs, allpurinol, Wilson's disease, large doses of vitamin C, Fanconi's syndrome, xanthinuria

ACE = Angiotensin coverting enzyme; VLDL = very low density lipoprotein.

APPENDIX-X

OTHER USEFUL TABLES

1(a) Recommended schedule for active immunization and skin testing of children

Age	Product administered	Test recommended
2 months	DTP, OPV, HbCV	
6 months	DTP, OPV, HbCV	
12 months	Measles-mumps-rubella	
15-19 months	DTP, OPV, MMR	Tuberculin test
4-6 years	DTP, OPV	Tuberculin test
11-12 years	Measles-mumps-rubella	Tuberculin test
14-16 years	Td (see comment)	

DTP = Diphtheria & tetanus toxoids with pertussis vaccine
OPV = Oral poliovirus vaccine containing attenuated poliovirus types 1, 2, and 3 (trivalent).
HbCV = Haemophilus *b* conjugate vaccine
MMR = Measles-Mumps-Rubella
Td = Adult tetanus toxoid (full dose) and diphtheria toxoid (reduced dose) for adult use. Repeat every 7-10 years.

1(b) Routine immunization for adults

Vaccine	Dose	Indications	Precautions
MMR	0.5 mL s.c. initially and at entry to college, military, etc.	Anyone born after 1956 and never infected or who is likely to be exposed	Do not give to pregnant women or to persons allergic to either egg protein or neomycin.
Td	0.5 mL IM initially, at 1 mo, after 6 mo, and q 10 yr	Anyone who has never been vaccinated should have primary series, followed by booster q 10 yr	Do not give to pregnant women or to persons allergic to horse serum
HB	1.0 mL IM initially, at 1 mo, and at 6 mo	Anyone likely to have any chance of an exposure	-
Influenza	0.5 mL IM	Medical personnel, persons desiring vaccination	Do not give to anyone with high fever or those allergic to egg protein

Pneumococcal	0.5 mL IM or s.c.	Anyone at high risk for pneumococcal disease	Do not give to pregnant women

MMR = Measles, Mumps, Rubella; HB=Hepatitis B; Td = Tetanus & Diphtheria toxoid.

1(c) Vaccines by type and recommended routes of administration

Vaccine	Type	Route
BCG	Live bacteria	Intradermal or s.c.
Cholera	Inactivated bacteria	Intradermal, IM or s.c.
DTP	Toxoids & inact. Bacteria	IM
HB	Inactive viral antigen	IM
Influenza	Inactive virus	IM
IPV	Inactivated virus	s.c.
Measles	Live virus	s.c.
MMR	Live viruses	s.c.
Mumps	Live virus	s.c.
OPV	Live viruses	Oral
Plague	Inactivated baceria	IM
Pneumococcal	Bacterial polysaccharides	IM or s.c.
Rabies	Inactivated virus	Intradermal or s.c.
Rubella	Live virus	s.c.
Tetanus	Inactivated toxin	IM
Td or DT	Inactivated toxins	IM
Typhoid	Inactivated bacteria Live attenuated vaccine	s.c. Oral
Yellow fever	Live virus	s.c.

BCG = Bacille Calmette-Guerin; DTP = Diphtheria, Tetanus, Pertussis
HB = Hepatitis B; IPV = Inactivated Poliovirus vaccine
OPV = Oral Poliovirus vaccine; Td = Tetanus & Diphtheria vaccine for use in persons over 7 years; DT = Diphtheria & Tetanus vaccine for use in children under 7 years; IM = Intramuscular; s.c. = Subcutaneous

2. The Apgar Score

Criteria	Score		
	0	1	2
Colour	Blue, pale	Body pink, Extremities blue	All pink
Heart rate	Absent	Below 100	Over 100

Respiration	Absent	Irregular, slow	Good, crying
Reflex response to nose catheter	None	Grimace	Sneeze, cough
Muscle tone	Limp	Some flexion of extremities	Active

Note : The *Apgar* scoring system estimates the severity of respiratory and neurologic depression at birth by rating certain signs. Every infant should be rated at exactly 1 and 5 minutes after birth, and both scores should be recorded. The maximum score of 10 is rare; the lower the score, the more severly depressed is the infant (Less than 5 indicates severe depression). Low scores are more likely to be associated with residual neurological damage or neonatal death, although most of these infants will survive and be normal.

3. The Glasgow Coma Score

Criteria	Score
Eyes open	
Never	1
To pain	2
To verbal stimuli	3
Spontaneously	4
Best verbal response	
No response	1
Incomprehensible sound	2
Inappropriate words	3
Disoriented and converses	4
Oriented and converses	5
Best motor response	
No response	1
Extension (decerebrate rigidity)	2
Flexion abnormal (decorticate rigidity)	3
Flexion withdrawal	4
Localized pain	5
Obeys	6
TOTAL :	3-15

Note : When carried out initially, the scale gives a rough indication of severity of brain injury. Coma grades 3 to 5 indicate potentially fatal damage, especially if accompanied by fixed pupils or absent oculovestibular responses. Conversely, admission scores of 8 or above correlate with a high chance of good recovery.

4. Blood and blood gases (normal values)

Category	*Normal values*
O_2 content	$\frac{(Hb \times 13.6 \times saturation\%)}{100} + (PO_2 \times 0.0031)$
Arterial saturation	95%
Pulmonary arterial O_2 saturation	75-80%
Whole blood O_2 capacity	17-21 mL of O_2/dL of blood
Arterial O_2 content	16-20 mL/dL of blood
Mixed venous O_2 content	10-16 mL/dL of blood
*p*H (arterial plasma)	7.39 – 7.41
CO_2 combining power (venous plasma)	21-30 mEq/L
Arterial CO_2 content (whole blood)	20-25 mEq/L
Arterial & alveolar CO_2 tension	37-41 mm Hg

5. (a) Tooth Eruption times

Deciduous teeth* (20 in number)	No.	Time of Eruption@ (in months)	Permanent teeth (32 in number)	No.	Time of Eruption@ (in years)
Lower central incisors	2	5-9	1st molars#	4	5-7
Upper central incisors	2	8-12	Incisors	8	6-8
Upper lateral incisors	2	10-12	Bicuspids	8	9-12
Lower lateral incisors	2	12-15	Canines	4	10-13
1st molars	4	10-16	2nd molars	4	11-14
Canines	4	16-20	3rd molars	4	17-25
2nd molars	4	20-30			

* The average child should have 6 teeth at age 1 yr., 12 teeth at 1.5 yr., 16 teeth at 2 yr., 20 teeth at 2.5 yr.

@ Varies greatly.

\# Molars are numbered from the front to the back of the mouth.

5. (b) Relationship between deciduous and permanent teeth*

20 Deciduous		32 Permanent	
Symbol	Name	Symbol	Name
A	Central incisor	1	Central incisor
B	Lateral incisor	2	Lateral incisor
C	Canine (cuspid)	3	Canine (cuspid)
D	1st molar	4	1st premolar (bicuspid)
E	2nd molar	5	2nd premolar (bicuspid)
		6	1st molar
		7	2nd molar
		8	3rd molar

* Each quadrant (left or right half of each jaw) contains the teeth listed.

5. (c) Shorthand representation of teeth

	Maxillary	
Right	─────┼─────	Left
	Mandibular	

Using the symbol for the tooth from Table 5(b)

⌈D represents the mandibular left deciduous 1st molar;

6⌋ represents the maxillary right permanent 1st molar.

6. Characteristics and reactions of the 4 blood types

ABO Types	Red Cells				Serum		
	Antigens present	Reactions with reagents			Antibodies present	Reaction with reagents	
		Anti A	Anti B	Anti A,B		A cells	B cells
O	Neither	–	–	–	Anti-A & B	+	+
A	A	+	–	+	Anti-B	–	+
B	B	–	+	+	Anti-A	+	–
AB	A and B	+	+	+	Neither	–	–

7. Standard basal metabolic rates

Weight (kg.)	Kcal/24 hours		
	Male	Both Sexes	Females
3		140	
5		270	
7		400	
9		500	
11		600	
13		650	
15		710	
17		780	
19		830	
21		880	
25	1020		960

Weight (kg.)	Kcal/24 hours		
	Male	Both Sexes	Females
29	1120		1040
33	1210		1120
37	1300		1190
41	1350		1260
45	1410		1320
49	1470		1380
53	1530		1440
57	1590		1500
61	1640		1560

Increments or decrements :

1. Add or subtract 12% of above for each degree C (8% for each degree F) above or below rectal temperature of 37.8 °C (100 °F).
2. Add 0-30% increments for usual activity; hypo- or hypermetabolic states require greater adjustments.

8. Risk of having a liveborn child with Down Syndrome or other chromosome abnormality.

Maternal Age	Risk of Down Syndrome	Total Risk for Chromosome abnormalities
20	1/1667	1/526
22	1/1429	1/500
24	1/1250	1/476
26	1/1176	1/455
28	1/1053	1/435
30	1/952	1/384
32	1/769	1/323
34	1/500	1/280
36	1/294	1/156
38	1/175	1/102
40	1/106	1/66
42	1/64	1/42
44	1/38	1/26
46	1/23	1/16
48	1/14	1/10
50	1/10	1/8

9. Some rough and ready rules

1. Weight in kg = (Age in years + 3) × 2.5

2. Length in cm

At birth	50 cm (± 3 cm)
1 year	75 cm (± 4 cm)
4 years	100 cm (± 5 cm)
7 years	125 cm (± 8 cm)
12 years	150 cm (± 10 cm)

3. Skull circumference in cm

At birth	
Pre-term	28-33
Term	35 (± 2 cm)
3 months	40
9 months	45
3 years	50
16 years	55

4. Surface area in m^2 (age in years + 6) × 7

5. Per cent of adult dose (weight in kg × 1.5) + 10

6. Per cent of adult dose (age in years × 4) + 20

10. Conversion Tables

(a) Fahrehheit-Celsius (Centigrade) Temperature Conversion

°F		°C
90	=	32.2
91	=	32.8
92	=	33.3
93	=	33.9
94	=	34.4
95	=	35.0
96	=	35.6
97	=	36.1
98	=	36.7
99	=	37.2
100	=	37.8
101	=	38.3

102	=	38.9
103	=	39.4
104	=	40.0
105	=	40.6
106	=	41.1
107	=	41.7
108	=	42.2
109	=	42.8

Conversion :

(i) To convert °F to °C subtract 32, then multiply by 5/9 or 0.555
(C = 5/9 [F – 32])

(ii) To convert °C to °F, multiply by 9/5 or 1.8, then add 32
(F = 9/5C + 32)

(b) Household Metric-Nonmetric Equivalents

1 Teaspoon (tsp)	=	5 mL
1 Tablespoon (tbsp)	=	15 mL = ½ fluid oz
1 Ounce (oz), fluid	=	30 mL
1 Ounce (oz), wt.	=	8.35 g
1 Cup	=	8 fl. Oz = 240 mL
1 Quart	=	946 mL
1 Pint	=	473 mL
1 Grain (gr)	=	65 mg

(c) Pounds to Kilograms (1kg = 2.2 : 1 lb = 0.45 kg)

lb	kg	lb	kg	lb	kg	lb	kg	lb	kg
5	2.3	50	22.7	95	43.1	140	63.5	185	83.9
10	4.5	55	25.0	100	45.4	145	65.8	190	86.2
15	6.8	60	27.2	105	47.6	150	68.0	195	88.5
20	9.1	65	29.5	110	49.9	155	70.3	200	90.7
25	11.3	70	31.7	115	52.2	160	72.6	205	93.0
30	13.6	75	34.0	120	54.4	165	74.8	210	95.3
35	15.9	80	36.3	125	56.7	170	77.1	215	97.5
40	18.1	85	38.6	130	58.9	175	79.4	220	99.8
45	20.4	90	40.8	135	61.2	180	81.6		

(d) Feet and Inches to Centimetres (1cm = 0.39 in : 1 in = 2.54 cm)

ft	in	cm	ft	in	cm	ft	in	cm	ft	in	cm	ft	in	cm
0	6	15.2	2	4	71.1	3	4	101.6	4	4	132.0	5	4	162.6
1	0	30.5	2	5	73.6	3	5	104.1	4	5	134.6	5	5	165.1
1	6	45.7	2	6	76.1	3	6	106.6	4	6	137.1	5	6	167.6
1	7	48.3	2	7	78.7	3	7	109.2	4	7	139.6	5	7	170.2
1	8	50.8	2	8	81.2	3	8	111.7	4	8	142.2	5	8	172.7
1	9	53.3	2	9	83.8	3	9	114.2	4	9	144.7	5	9	175.3
1	10	55.9	2	10	86.3	3	10	116.8	4	10	147.3	5	10	177.8
1	11	58.4	2	11	88.8	3	11	119.3	4	11	149.8	5	11	180.3
2	0	61.0	3	0	91.4	4	0	121.9	5	0	152.4	6	0	182.9
2	1	63.5	3	1	93.9	4	1	124.4	5	1	154.9	6	1	185.4
2	2	66.0	3	2	96.4	4	2	127.0	5	2	157.5	6	2	188.0
2	3	68.6	3	3	99.0	4	3	129.5	5	3	160.0	6	3	190.5

11. Desirable Weights (in Pounds)

Men (Age 25 and Over)				Women (Age 25 and Over)**			
Height* Ft. In.	Small Frame	Medium Frame	Large Frame	Height* Ft. In.	Small Frame	Medium Frame	Large Frame
5 2	112-120	118-129	126-141	4 10	92-98	96-107	104-119
5 3	115-123	121-133	129-144	4 11	94-101	98-110	106-122
5 4	118-126	124-136	132-148	5 0	96-104	101-113	109-125
5 5	121-129	127-139	135-152	5 1	99-107	104-116	112-128
5 6	124-133	130-143	138-156	5 2	102-110	107-119	115-131
5 7	128-137	134-147	142-161	5 3	105-113	110-122	118-134
5 8	132-141	138-152	147-166	5 4	108-116	113-126	121-138
5 9	136-145	142-156	151-170	5 5	111-119	116-130	125-142
5 10	140-150	146-160	155-174	5 6	114-123	120-135	129-146
5 11	144-154	150-165	159-179	5 7	118-127	124-139	133-150
6 0	148-158	154-170	164-184	5 8	121-131	128-143	137-154
6 1	152-162	158-175	168-189	5 9	126-135	132-147	141-158
6 2	156-167	162-180	173-194	5 10	130-140	136-151	145-163
6 3	160-171	167-185	178-199	5 11	134-144	140-155	149-168
6 4	164-175	172-190	182-204	6 0	138-148	144-159	153-173

* With shoes with 1-inch heels.

* With shoes with 2-inch heels

** For women between 18 and 25, subtract 1 lb for each year under 25.

BIBLIOGRAPHY

Allaby, M. *Dictionary of the Environment.* London Press, Southampton, 1975.

Armitage, P. *Statistical Methods in Medical Research.* Blackwell, Oxford, 1971.

Borders, R.J. *The Dictionary of Health Physics & Nuclear Sciences Terms.* RSA Publications, Hebron, 1991.

Bowman, W.C. *Dictionary of Pharmacology.* Blackwell, London, 1986.

Colton, T. *Statistics in Medicine,* Little, Brown; Boston, 1974.

Dupayarat, J. *Dictionary of Biomedical Acronyms and Abbreviations.* Wiley, New York, 1990.

Fairpo, J.E.H. and Fairpo, C.G. *Heinemann Dental Dictionary.* Heinemann, London, 1987.

Farr, A.D. (Ed). *Dictionary of Medical Laboratory Sciences.* Blackwell, London, 1988.

Farrell, T.K. *The Glossary of Optical Terminology.* Fairchild Publications, New York, 1986.

Fay, J.F. *The Alcohol/Drug Dictionary and Encyclopaedia,* C.C. Thomas, Springfield, Ill, 1988.

Froom, J. *An International Glossary for Primary Care.* J. Family Pract., 13: 673 – 681, 1981.

Goodwin, D.M. *A Dictionary of Neuropsychology.* Springer-Verlag, New York, 1989.

Hanken, M.A. and Water, K.A. (Eds). *Glossary of Healthcare Terms.* AHIMA, Chicago, 1994.

Herbert, W.J., Wilkinson, P.C., and Stott, D.I. *Dictionary of Immunology.* Blackwell, Oxford, 1985.

Hodgson, B., Mailman, R.B., and Chambers, J.E. *Macmillan Dictionary of Toxicology.* Macmillan, London, 1988.

Hogarth, J. *Glossary of Health Care Terminology.* W.H.O., Copenhagen, 1982.

Note : Many of the works on this list, contain glossaries, and nearly all contain definitions that have been adapted and included in this dictionary.

Kendall, M.G., Buckland, A.A. *A Dictionary of Statistical Terms.* London, Longman, 1982.

Last, J.M., (Ed). *A Dictionary of Epidemiology.* Oxford University Press, New York, 1988.

Lindsay, M.P. *Dictionary of Mental Handicaps.* Routledge, London, 1989.

Lynch M. (Ed). *Health Insurance Terminology.* Health Insurance Institute of Washington, D.C., 1992.

Meadows, A.J., Gordon, M., and Singleton, A. *A Dictionary of New Information Technology.* Century. London, 1982.

Millodot, M. *Dictionary of Optometry.* Butterworths, London, 1986.

National Governor's Association. *Glossary of Health Insurance Terms.* N.G.A., Washington D.C., 1992.

Pressat, R. *Dictionary of Demography.* Blackwell, Oxford, 1985.

Reiger, R., Michaelis, A. and Green M.M. *Glossary of Genetics.* Springer-Verlag, New York, 1991.

Skinner, H.A. *The Origin of Medical Terms.* Williams & Wilkins, Baltimore, 1961.

Slee, V.N. and Slee, D.A. *Health Care Terms.* Tringa Press, St. Paul, Minnesota, 1993.

Smith, B.C. and Smith, B.E. *Medical Terminology for the Health Professions.* Harcourt Brace Jovanovich, Chicago, 1986.

Sohm, E.D. (Ed). *Glossary of Evaluation Terms.* United Nations, Geneva, 1978.

Susser, M.W., Watson, W. Hopper K. *Sociology in Medicine.* Oxford University Press, New York, 1985.

Timmreck, T. *Dictionaty of Health Services Management.* Rynd Communications, Washington, 1987.

United Health Corp. *The Managed Care Resource: The Language of Managed Health Care.* Minnetonka, Minn., U.H.C.C., 1992.

Walton, H. (Ed). *Dictionary of Psychiatry.* Blackwell, London, 1985.

West, G.P. (Ed). *Black's Veterinary Dictionary.* A&C Black, London,1995.

World Bank. *A Glossary of Population Terminology.* Washington: World Bank, Washington, 1985.

World Health Organization. *Glossary of Terms.* W.H.O. Geneva, 1984.